Mind
Your Gut

Also by Kate Scarlata:

The Low-FODMAP Diet Step by Step:

A Personalized Plan to Relieve the Symptoms of IBS

21-Day Tummy: The Revolutionary Diet that Sooths and

Shrinks any Belly Fast

Mind
Your Gut

THE SCIENCE-BASED, WHOLE-BODY GUIDE TO LIVING WELL WITH IBS

KATE SCARLATA, MPH, RDN, AND **MEGAN RIEHL**, PSYD

Foreword by WILLIAM D. CHEY, MD

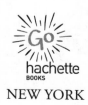

hachette
BOOKS

NEW YORK

Copyright © 2024 by Kate Scarlata and Megan E. Riehl
Cover design by Terri Sirma
Jacket images © ridhobadal/Shutterstock
Cover copyright © 2024 by Hachette Book Group, Inc.

Hachette Go, an imprint of Hachette Books
Hachette Book Group
1290 Avenue of the Americas
New York, NY 10104
HachetteGo.com
Facebook.com/HachetteGo
Instagram.com/HachetteGo

First Edition: March 2024

Published by Hachette Go, an imprint of Hachette Book Group, Inc.
The Hachette Go name and logo is a trademark of the Hachette Book Group.

The Hachette Speakers Bureau provides a wide range of authors for speaking events. To find out more, go to hachettespeakersbureau.com or email HachetteSpeakers@hbgusa.com.

Hachette Go books may be purchased in bulk for business, educational, or promotional use. For information, please contact your local bookseller or Hachette Book Group Special Markets Department at: special.markets@hbgusa.com.

The publisher is not responsible for websites (or their content) that are not owned by the publisher.

Print book interior design by Bart Dawson.

Library of Congress Cataloging-in-Publication Data has been applied for.

ISBNs: 978-0-306-83233-8 (hardcover); 978-0-306-83235-2 (ebook)

Printed in the United States of America

LSC-C

Printing 1, 2023

We dedicate this book to any person living with IBS who will not settle for a treatment plan that prevents them from living fully. We are grateful to our patients past, present, and future. It is truly our honor to contribute to your care and well-being.

"You can't stop the waves, but you can learn to surf."

—Jon Kabat-Zinn

CONTENTS

FOREWORD

William D. Chey, MD, Chief of Gastroenterology,
Michigan Medicine

What a long, strange trip it's been." This classic line from the Grateful Dead describes the evolution of treating irritable bowel syndrome, or IBS, over the last seven decades. Early on, the prevailing wisdom held that IBS was a manifestation of psychiatric disease. A friend and colleague of mine, who went to medical school in the 1960s, recalled a lecture in which the professor alluded to the pathophysiology of IBS by describing the gastrointestinal tract as "the playground of a disturbed mind." This brand of thinking enabled years of stigma, delegitimization, lack of empathy, and misguided attributions of "it's all in your head."

Fortunately, in recent years an array of more scientific explanations for symptoms in patients with IBS has emerged. These include abnormalities in how the GI tract moves, hyperactive sensation in the bowel, genetic factors, and abnormalities in the bowel environment. These are affected by the food we eat, the various organisms that live in the gut (gut microbiota), and the many different substances (e.g., bile acids and neurotransmitters) that are released into the lining of the gut. In fact, there is a gut-brain connection, as the gut wall has a nervous system, called the enteric nervous system. Recent work has found that the degree to which this microenvironment can activate the immune system and the enteric nervous system is dependent on the permeability of the cells lining the small intestine and colon.

All these different concepts strongly suggest that IBS isn't a single disease. IBS is likely composed of a number of different diseases that present with similar symptoms, and for which we currently do not have reliable diagnostic tests that can separate patients on the basis of the specific cause of their symptoms. The fact that IBS isn't a single disease explains why there is no silver-bullet treatment. Patients and providers alike are frustrated by the fact that most IBS medications improve selected symptoms in only half or fewer of patients treated. This doesn't mean that the medications don't work. In fact, high-quality clinical trials show they do work better than placebo. However, if we understand that IBS isn't one disease, it begins to make more sense that no single drug will make all patients, or even a majority, better. Again, that's not to say that medications don't have an important role to play in the treatment of IBS symptoms. They do. Medications are often *part of* the solution—but not *the* solution—for patients with this vexing condition.

The vast majority of patients with IBS associate their symptoms with two key triggers: food and stress. As it turns out, a diet low in certain sugars—called fermentable oligosaccharides, disaccharides, monosaccharides, and polyols (aka FODMAPs)—can help improve IBS symptoms. This diet was first described and validated by investigators at Monash University in Australia. Their research inspired the creation of our GI nutrition program at the University of Michigan in 2007. At that time, GI nutrition as a specialty was in its infancy, and I am proud to say that ours was one of the first programs at a major US medical center. We had to scratch and claw for resources, let alone credibility with our own doctors.

Shortly after starting the program, I was invited to deliver a lecture on IBS at an annual meeting of the American College of

Gastroenterology. I used the occasion to introduce the thousands of mainstream gastroenterologists in attendance to the low-FODMAP diet as a treatment option. At the time, the data supporting the low-FODMAP diet for IBS was sparse, so I anticipated some level of controversy. Well, let's just say that my instincts proved correct. Most of the feedback fell between curious skepticism and outright anger that I would amplify this radical concept by discussing it in such a high-profile forum. Yet, among the many skeptics, there were notable exceptions. In particular, two dietitians made their way to the podium after my talk and thanked me for acknowledging the importance of foods as a trigger for patients with IBS. I was fascinated to hear they had been using the low-FODMAP diet in their private practice with a great deal of success. One of those dietitians was Kate Scarlata. Though she was not well known in medical circles at the time, her support and advocacy for patients with IBS and for dietitians with an interest in IBS helped spawn the specialty of GI nutrition. Over the last fourteen years, we have worked closely together, and now, a speaker would be remiss to deliver a lecture about IBS at a national meeting without discussing dietary interventions.

What about addressing the influence of stress on IBS? Given the success of our nutrition program, in 2014 we set out to build a GI behavioral health program to complement it. I called my good friend and colleague Dr. Laurie Keefer, who had built one of the first and most successful GI behavioral health programs in the United States at Northwestern University. As fate would have it, Laurie was training a clinical psychologist named Megan Riehl, who was eager to help build and lead a program at Michigan. At the time, there were fewer than a dozen well-trained GI psychologists in the entire United States. Thanks to Megan, today we have one of the most respected GI behavioral health programs in the country. In addition, she leads one of the only postdoctoral training programs in GI behavioral health in the world.

I give you this background to certify that Kate and Megan are the real deal. They are not just experts—they helped *create* and *shape* their respective fields. They bring all their experience to bear in *Mind Your Gut*. The book rightfully presents food and stress as codependent influences in the pathogenesis and treatment of IBS. I am confident that the strategies in this book will help you be more confident in managing your IBS, enabling you to take back control of your life.

INTRODUCTION

We are honored to share with you our strategies developed from years of working with individuals living with irritable bowel syndrome (IBS). This disorder can be frustrating, even devastating, and we enthusiastically conceived of this book out of our desire to provide life-changing care for anyone who has not yet had adequate relief of their symptoms. Working in concert with a skilled gastroenterologist, we like to call our combined expertise—that of a registered dietitian and a GI psychologist—the Dream Team model. With the Dream Team approach, you get the best of all worlds: a holistic toolbox of proven skills and resources that we each use daily in our clinical practices. For many people, access to a Dream Team approach has been difficult to find. One survey conducted by the International Foundation for Functional Gastrointestinal Disorders (IFFGD) in collaboration with experts from the University of North Carolina found that being diagnosed with IBS took on average 6.6 years after symptoms began, leaving individuals with IBS to suffer without targeted treatments to provide symptom relief. We were motivated to change that with *Mind Your Gut*.

In this book, we'll take you on a deep dive into the inner workings of the brain and gut. We'll show you how simple changes to behavior and nutrition can be powerful ways to improve your IBS, and how you can adapt the tools we provide to create your own personalized program toward living better with IBS. We start off in Chapter 1 with an introduction to IBS and how food and mental health can make symptoms better or worse. We address the brain-gut connection in Chapters 2–4, moving through science-based strategies for behavioral change. In Chapters 5–7 we describe the nutritional aspects of IBS, explaining how and why certain foods can trigger gut symptoms. We also delve into the importance of having a healthy relationship with food despite this illness, along with the risks of overly restricting one's diet. In Chapter 8 we break down the key aspects of the gut microbiome—a new and interesting field—detailing how the tiny microbes that inhabit your gut relate to IBS and offering tips to promote your gut health for the long haul.

Are intestinal pain and diarrhea your main problems? Constipation? We've got you covered. Since IBS is a symptom-based diagnosis, in Chapter 9 we delve into symptom-based solutions with a full toolkit of treatments backed by science. And although an IBS diagnosis is typically spot-on, other conditions may mimic IBS or overlap with it. In Chapter 10 we run through these to provide all the information you need so you can discuss any concerns you may have with your treatment team.

The last section of the book contains a gold mine of resources that you can tailor to your own needs, including food brands we love, how to select a probiotic supplement, how to access health professionals to guide your personal treatment, our favorite digital therapeutics, helpful websites, and so much more. Throughout the book, you will find sidebars like the Gut Game Changer, which highlights key gut-health topics and busts myths; the Brain Bite, which features brain-gut related topics; and the Digestible Detail, which highlights important nutrition concepts.

In our collective clinical experience, we have provided care to a diverse group of patients of all ages, utilizing our science-based methods to help them move forward from debilitating symptoms to engaging in full lives. Our patients have included college students with perfectionistic tendencies leading to major tummy troubles at exam time, early career professionals trying to establish themselves without the stress of IBS, athletes hoping to embark on their first marathon without having to drop out of the race due to an unruly gut, women wanting to conceive their first child but afraid of how their gut will respond, and adventurous retirees yearning to freely plan dream vacations. A holistic and integrative approach to the management of IBS can be life-changing. This is the book, we are your team, and we welcome you. Get ready to be empowered to mind your gut!

CHAPTER 1

IBS: THE GUT, BRAIN, AND FOOD CONNECTION

Holding this book is an indicator that you are looking for change. No doubt you are tired of the abdominal pain, bloating, diarrhea, or constipation—or all of the above—that's wreaking havoc on your health, not to mention the other areas of your life. Does it seem like you spend a good part of your day thinking about food and what you can eat to keep your gut symptoms in check? Have you avoided eating until later in the day—otherwise you would be in the bathroom so long that you'd be late for school or work? Are you pulling back from traveling with family and friends because of the fear your gut will get out of whack? Does anticipation of gut symptoms stop you in your tracks when you have a big event at work or with friends? Does experiencing a cleansing poop seem impossible or take much longer than you hoped? The constellation of symptoms that makes up irritable bowel syndrome (IBS)

is unfortunately extremely common. But there is hope. We are so glad you are here, because within these pages are solutions. You'll find ways to improve your digestive symptoms that are sustainable and backed by science. In the world of IBS management, science has confirmed that patients who utilize a team-based approach—with experts in medical management, nutrition, and behavioral health—have the greatest opportunities for improvement. It's your turn to feel better now. Welcome to the team!

IBS EXPLAINED

What is IBS, anyway? Let's take a closer look at this often-misunderstood condition. IBS is a chronic and often debilitating gastrointestinal (GI) disorder characterized by abdominal pain and a change in bowel habits. The pain experienced in IBS is often described as cramping with variable intensity that flares frequently. It's the most common reason to seek help from a gastroenterologist, accounting for up to 50 percent of GI doctor visits. If you have IBS (or suspect that you might), you're certainly not alone. IBS afflicts about 11 percent of the global population and about forty-five million people in the United States. More than twice as many women as men are diagnosed with IBS, and it most often affects people between twenty and thirty years old.

ROME IV IBS DIAGNOSTIC CRITERIA

A reliable IBS diagnosis can be made by your gastroenterologist when features such as blood in the stool, weight loss, nocturnal (while sleeping) symptoms, a family history of colon cancer, and anemia have been ruled out and your symptoms fulfill the following IBS criteria by the Rome Foundation, a nonprofit organization founded to help people with GI disorders:

Recurrent abdominal pain on average at least one day per week in the last three months, associated with **two or more** of the following criteria:*

1. Related to defecation
2. Associated with a change in frequency of stool
3. Associated with a change in form (appearance) of stool

* Criteria fulfilled for the last three months with symptom onset at least six months prior to diagnosis.

Depending on its most prevalent symptom, IBS is grouped into subtypes, including IBS with diarrhea (IBS-D), IBS with constipation (IBS-C), and IBS with mixed bowel patterns (IBS-M). Additionally, after an episode of acute gastroenteritis (such as the result of food poisoning), postinfectious IBS (PI-IBS) may be diagnosed in individuals who previously did not have IBS but meet the criteria after the infection. Of note, PI-IBS occurs more frequently in women, in those exposed to antibiotics, and in patients who have a history of anxiety or depression.

DRIVING FACTORS BEHIND AN IBS DIAGNOSIS

IBS doesn't have a single cause. The condition often results from a variety of factors that affect gut function, the inner workings of the brain, and more. There are known environmental triggers of IBS, such as stressors, food intolerances, antibiotic use, and previous episodes of gastroenteritis, for example, from foodborne illness. In fact, infectious gastroenteritis is the strongest risk factor for later developing IBS. Genetics may also play a role, as biological family members of people with the disorder have been shown to have an increased risk.

COMMON IBS SCENARIOS: CAN YOU RELATE?

While each pathway to IBS is unique, there are some common scenarios associated with the onset of symptoms. Understanding these may help inform your personal roadmap to improvement. See if your history resembles any of these examples.

CHILDHOOD TUMMY TROUBLES (GENETICS AT PLAY)

"I was born this way. I've just always had stomach issues."
"My mother tells me that from the beginning I was allergic to formula."
"As a kid, I was told not to complain and to just shake it off."
"I never knew that fairly constant abdominal pain and going days without a bowel movement wasn't normal. We never talked about it in my family."

DIETARY INTOLERANCES (NUTRITION OR POSSIBLE GUT-MICROBIOME-RELATED RISKS)

"I was a picky eater as a child."
"I was diagnosed with severe lactose intolerance at one year old."
"I never know what foods might trigger my symptoms."

I WAS PERFECTLY HEALTHY UNTIL . . . (POSTINFECTIOUS)

"I went out of the country on vacation and got sick. It's like I never got better."
"I had a bad bout of gastroenteritis and was prescribed several rounds of antibiotics."
"I experienced food poisoning after ordering dinner out of a food truck, and now I can't eat anything."

THE MESS OF STRESS (PSYCHOSOCIAL FACTORS)

"My symptoms are the worst before a big exam or presentation."

"I planned my entire wedding, made it through the day, and spent my entire honeymoon in the bathroom."

"My life and my work revolve around my bowels. I can't have morning meetings, and the thought of work travel is debilitating."

HIDDEN EFFECTS OF TRAUMA (POST-TRAUMATIC STRESS)

"My childhood was chaotic to say the least, and I was a kid with constant stomachaches."

"I was raped at the age of fifteen. But I didn't have GI symptoms like this until I was much older."

"My family came to the US from Iraq after the war. I don't remember having symptoms before coming to the US."

IBS presents with abnormal intestinal movements, a heightened sense of pain in the gut (formally known as visceral hypersensitivity), and dysregulation of the gut-brain axis, a bidirectional communication pathway between the gut and brain. In IBS, the shift in how the gut and brain communicate is a central feature. It's as if the gut and brain are not talking to each other but rather screaming with a megaphone. IBS also often coexists with anxiety and depression, as well as a GI-specific type of anxiety known as visceral anxiety (worry about your GI symptoms). In fact, this GI-specific anxiety can cause people who live with IBS to unnecessarily avoid certain foods.

Unsurprisingly, at the microscopic level, the gut of an IBS patient often looks different from a healthy gut. Mast cells, a type of immune system cell, have been shown to be higher in number or to be more reactive in many people with IBS—sometimes both. The highly reactive intestinal mast cells in IBS appear to contribute significantly to abdominal pain. Interestingly, both diet and stress can activate the mast cells—and this may be one reason why lifestyle therapies offer IBS patients relief from symptoms.

GETTING DIAGNOSED

When you have physical GI symptoms, the first step toward changing the trajectory of your health is to see a medical doctor. Since IBS symptoms can mimic many other medical issues, including potentially life-threatening ones like colon cancer and ovarian cancer, *it is imperative that you don't self-diagnose yourself with IBS.* The internet is a great tool for all of us, but it shouldn't be used as a substitute for a professional assessment of your health.

Your physician may ask you to provide information about what lands in your toilet using a visual guide such as the Bristol Stool Form Scale, which helps gather information about the consistency, texture, and shape of your stool (see page 319 in the Resources to find this helpful tool). After the physical exam, your physician will analyze your symptoms along with your medical and family history and may order lab tests to help guide the correct diagnosis and treatment plan. Always consult your doctor to assess your symptoms and receive a proper diagnosis.

WHAT KIND OF MEDICAL PROVIDERS DO YOU NEED?

A family medicine or primary care doctor can make a diagnosis of IBS after an initial consultation, physical exam, and some preliminary testing. They may also refer you to a gastroenterologist for further testing. Gastroenterologists specialize in the therapeutic management and diagnosis of IBS, which may include performing a colonoscopy if you need one, prescribing medication, or referring you to other providers, such as a GI dietitian or GI psychologist.

If you are newly diagnosed or an individual with IBS that is poorly controlled, the next step in your treatment is to take a Dream Team approach. As the field of gastroenterology evolves, we are learning that one provider alone is rarely able to meet the unique needs of someone living with IBS. Further, we all have some forms of stress in our lives, and for people with IBS, simply eating can be one of those stressors. A GI dietitian can help you discover how a nutrition tune-up and plan can help you manage food-related digestive distress. Your personalized IBS treatment plan may also include working with a GI psychologist or mental health expert who specializes in the management of GI conditions. They will help you gain insights into how life events and stress can affect the way your brain and gut communicate. Brain-gut behavioral therapies rework how you think about your symptoms and improve your ability to manage them. Recent science has shown that working with an integrated team of IBS experts (a GI registered dietitian, a GI psychologist, and a gastroenterologist), versus a gastroenterologist alone, results in better clinical management and reduced costs. Unfortunately, not everyone has access to a Dream Team due to lack of expert GI dietitians and psychologists in their geographic area, poor insurance coverage, and other inequities that are common in our medical system. This situation prompted our desire to write this book. We wanted to improve access to our tried-and-true scientific approaches.

Here are some questions that may help you determine where you have been and what you want to try next. In the initial consultation with a new provider, the following topics will be discussed. You might find it helpful to jot down your answers prior to your initial appointment.

- When did your GI symptoms begin?
- How long have you been experiencing GI distress?
- What kind of medical workup have you had?
- Do you have a diagnosis from a medical professional?
- What have you been told about your diagnosis (treatment plan, expectations for improvements, etc.)?
- What has helped your symptoms (medications, stress management, diet changes, etc.)?

- What has made your symptoms worse (stress, certain foods, other health issues, etc.)?
- Describe your relationship with food.
- Do you think about food most of the day?
- Do your food-related symptoms limit your ability to eat at a restaurant or at a friend's home?

Each provider on your GI care team will support your total health needs while you explore treatments to figure out what helps you best mitigate your gut symptoms. Check out the Resources to help you find suitable IBS experts (such as a gastroenterologist, GI dietitian, GI psychologist, and more) to work with. They can help maximize your health and provide you with the support you need to fully manage your GI symptoms.

THE IBS MEDICAL WORKUP: UNTANGLING THE COMPLEXITY OF GI DISTRESS

For IBS symptoms (abdominal pain, cramping, bloating, diarrhea, and/or constipation), the medical workup often begins with blood work, stool tests, and perhaps a colonoscopy or endoscopy to rule out other conditions (see Table 1). Red-flag symptoms such as blood in the stool, weight loss, waking in the night with pain or diarrhea, or anemia will be assessed, as these are not attributable to IBS. If your family history includes inflammatory bowel disease, celiac disease, or GI malignancy, that will be considered as well, given the higher risk of these conditions for people with a family history of them.

Currently no tests have validated biomarkers (indicators) for IBS—meaning you won't have a test come back that says you're "positive" for IBS. Rather, a positive diagnosis is arrived at when your symptoms fit the Rome Foundation's criteria for IBS (see page 6), alarm features are not present (weight loss, blood in stool, nighttime symptoms), and clinical assessments provided by your gastroenterol-ogist (results from lab tests and other procedures such as a colonos-copy) have yielded negative results for certain other conditions.

GUT GAME CHANGER: BEWARE OF UNPROVEN IBS BIOMARKER TESTS

The existing blood test on the market for IBS is inadequate due to low sensitivity, meaning that it produces a high number of false negatives. According to current data, nearly half of individuals *with* IBS could have a negative test (i.e., the test tells you that you don't have IBS, but you do). Researchers are prioritizing the development of a reliable biomarker for IBS, but meanwhile, keep your money in your pocket until this testing evolves.

TABLE 1. COMMON INITIAL TESTS FOR AN IBS WORKUP

Complete blood count (CBC): A blood test helpful to evaluate your overall health and capable of detecting a wide range of disorders, such as anemia or infection.

C-reactive protein (CRP): A blood test to determine if there is inflammation somewhere in your body.

Tissue transglutaminase antibodies (tTG-IgA): A blood test to screen for celiac disease.

Immunoglobulin A, quantitative: A blood test to assess immunoglobulin A (IgA), an antibody blood protein that's part of your immune system. Your body makes IgA and other types of antibodies to help fight off infections. Quantitative IgA should be ordered along with the tTG-IgA, as a low level will affect the accuracy of this celiac disease marker.

Fecal calprotectin: A stool test to assess for elevation of neutrophils (white blood cells that help fight infection) in the intestinal mucosa, which occurs during intestinal inflammation. It can indicate a need for further testing for potential inflammatory bowel disease.

Colonoscopy: A flexible scope inserted via the rectum to detect changes or abnormalities in the large intestine.

In some instances, a more extensive workup may be ordered based on your physician's clinical judgment from the information gathered during your medical visit (see Table 2).

TABLE 2. ADDITIONAL TESTS THAT *MAY* BE CONSIDERED IN AN IBS WORKUP

Abdominal X-ray: An image of the abdomen to assess for excess stool or abnormalities in the intestine.

Endoscopy: A flexible scope inserted into the upper gastrointestinal tract to assess changes or abnormalities in the esophagus, stomach, and the beginning of the small intestine (duodenum).

Breath testing for lactose malabsorption (LM) or small intestinal bacterial overgrowth (SIBO). Breath testing is an indirect measure of gut microbial metabolism. In SIBO testing, lactulose or glucose is ingested; a subsequent rise of gas levels above normal criteria indicates a positive SIBO test. Higher than normal gas levels during this test reflect microbial production of gas (hydrogen, methane, and in some cases hydrogen sulfide). For LM testing, lactose is ingested. A subsequent rise in gas levels above normal criteria indicates LM.

Anal rectal manometry (ARM) or defecography assesses how effectively the rectum and anal sphincter are working together to eliminate feces.

Allergy testing: When symptoms beyond the GI tract such as hives or other allergic symptoms repeatedly occur with ingestion of food, allergy testing may be required. (Allergy risk in IBS is lower than food intolerance reactions, but allergies are on the rise.)

Gastric emptying testing measures whether the stomach empties normally, too quickly, or too slowly. When upper-GI symptoms such as fullness after eating, heartburn, or nausea occur along with bloating in the upper-GI tract, this test may be considered.

If persistent debilitating symptoms are not reduced after you and your treatment team have tried a number of therapies, take a peek at Chapters 9 and 10 for additional symptom-based treatment strategies as well as possible IBS mimickers to review with your providers.

A POSITIVE SPIN ON YOUR NEGATIVE WORKUP

When a lab test provides an objective positive result, this can begin to bring a certain amount of relief to a patient who has been suffering: "Now I finally know what is wrong!" However, when test after test comes back "normal," and you remain uncomfortable with GI distress or perhaps even notice you are getting worse, that relief can lead to concern: "Will they ever find out what is wrong with me?" We understand why you might feel this way. Remember, with IBS, your labs may come back normal despite your symptoms.

What happens next illustrates the importance of good provider and patient communication. Ideally, you would sit down with your medical provider to discuss what it means to have ongoing symptoms despite normal test results. In a perfect scenario, your doctor would look you in the eye with compassion and say something like this:

Your test results indicate that you do not have anything structurally abnormal. You do not have inflammatory bowel disease or cancer. What your symptoms indicate is that you have a diagnosis of irritable bowel syndrome, or IBS. It is a complex digestive condition that can occur due to a variety of factors. It can be triggered by stress, diet, and even unco-ordinated nerve and muscle function in your pelvic area that can benefit from physical therapy. I am going to help you manage these symptoms, and we will also discuss working with other specialists such as a registered dietitian, a mental health professional with expertise in GI conditions, and possibly a physical therapist. We will all work together to get you feeling better. I am confident that these treatments will be helpful!

Unfortunately, many patients have not had the Dream Team experience and instead hear something like this: "Good news, the workups are normal. You might have IBS, but there's not much that can be done about it." End of story.

Or a patient receives a brief message in their patient portal that says their tests are "unremarkable" or "benign," and otherwise never hears back from the provider.

Or—and we gulp and shake our heads when we hear this one—"It's just IBS. It's in your head." That one is a real kick in the stomach for someone suffering with life-altering intestinal pain. It can leave people feeling as though their medical provider doesn't understand or is dismissing the severity of their pain. You may worry something has been missed, because surely these physical symptoms are indic-ative of something wrong, or worse yet, that you are someone who just can't be helped. You're left without a clear roadmap for how to feel better, and the lack of empathy can lead to distrust toward the medical community and hopelessness. If you've received anything less than the Dream Team approach, this book will provide guidance and will empower you with information to advocate for your care, so you can get out of the bathroom and back on your feet.

THE SECOND BRAIN: UNDERSTANDING GUT FEELINGS

Your intestinal tract and your brain are connected—so much so that the gut can be thought of as a second brain. A fun fact: more than 90 percent of the body's serotonin and 50 percent of the body's dopamine—key neurotransmitters—are produced in the gut. It turns out we can give credence to the concept of trusting your gut instinct. Indeed, your gut is producing chemicals and sending signals to the big brain up top! Similarly, you are also getting feedback from your brain when you feel those butterflies in your stomach during periods of stress, excitement, or anxiety.

Though we all feel stress sometimes, the stress response in IBS is exaggerated. In the following chapters you will learn calming responses that can decrease GI distress in moments when they can be most helpful (e.g., before a big exam, a presentation, or travel). Before we dive into these strategies, let's learn a bit more about the bidirectional superhighway connecting the brain and gut. Put on your thinking cap—here's a quick science lesson about the nervous system.

Zooming out, your body's nervous system has two major parts, the central nervous system (CNS) and the peripheral nervous system (PNS). The CNS is composed of the brain and spinal cord. The PNS connects the CNS to the other parts of the body. The PNS carries messages back and forth between the brain and the organs and muscles.

The PNS has two key parts: the somatic nervous system, which controls voluntary processes, like moving your arm, and the autonomic nervous system, which controls unconscious processes. These unconscious processes are classified as either parasympathetic, like the heartbeat and digestive processes ("rest and digest"), or sympathetic, like the stress response ("fight or flight"). The gut's nervous system, called the enteric nervous system (ENS), is a main part of the autonomic nervous system and is often called the second brain.

The ENS has two branching networks of nerves known as the submucosal plexus and the myenteric plexus. The submucosal plexus controls gastric secretions, absorption, and muscle movements in the digestive tract. The myenteric plexus can increase tone of the gut, speed (motility), and intensity of the contractions that take place during the digestive process. Inhibition of the myenteric system helps relax the muscular rings (sphincters) that control the journey of digested food and waste.

The ENS lines your entire digestive tract, from mouth to anus, with millions of neurons that facilitate communication with the central nervous system. Interestingly, the ENS produces many of the same neurotransmitters that are produced in your CNS, such as dopamine, serotonin, and acetylcholine, all chemicals that play a big role in how you feel physically and emotionally.

Each person has a hardwired connection between the brain in the head (part of the CNS) and the ENS. This bidirectional pathway is known as the gut-brain axis (GBA). The ENS lives within the walls of the GI tract and communicates with the brain through the spinal cord. One more key element of this communication pathway are the vagal nerves, which line the parasympathetic nervous system within the ENS. Slow and deep breathing can stimulate the vagus nerve to induce the rest-and-digest response. The vagus nerve oversees crucial bodily functions, including mood, immune response, heart rate, and digestion. The CNS and ENS are derived from the same cells during fetal development, so it is no wonder they continue to work together and communicate directly with each other. Take a look at Figure 1 to see the effects of the bidirectional pathway that runs between the gut and brain.

HOW THE GUT AND BRAIN COMMUNICATE IN IBS

That's how the gut communicates in general. Now let's talk about what happens if someone has IBS. As mentioned, the stress response in IBS is exaggerated, and stress affects the digestive tract.

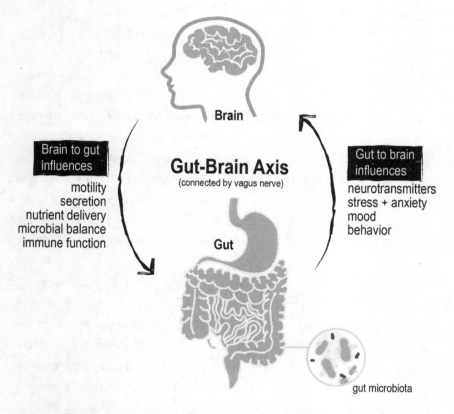

Figure 1. The Bidirectional Pathway of the Gut-Brain Axis

While the ENS typically operates the GI tract independently, the brain via the CNS can influence how it behaves. In fact, novel research has shown that specific parts of the brain that affect sensory processing, emotional regulation, and cognition are altered in the brain networks of people with IBS. Here lies the dilemma: the gut doesn't always seem to behave the way we'd like it to, but the brain is actively involved in this behavior. In times of stress, the ENS may send a distress signal that makes the GI system run differently. In IBS, stress can also make the nerves in the gut overly sensitive (known as visceral hypersensitivity), so sensations in the gut that most people would not feel might be perceived as unpleasant by a person with IBS.

HELLO, GUT, THIS IS YOUR BRAIN TALKING

Does it seem like your IBS acts up at the least convenient times? Like it somehow knows you have a plane to catch? That unease in your stomach may happen before a performance, an important meeting, a big exam, or even a party. Commonly this is followed by an urgent sensation that prompts a mad dash to the loo or sometimes may lead to an inability to poop. These sensations come on during periods of stress. Most people, even those without a digestive condition, can recall a few times in life when this has happened.

The sensation of butterflies in the stomach typically floats away as the perception of stress decreases and the individual can revert their attention back to the situation at hand. Their brain is no longer focusing on the happenings of the gut because it has other things to focus on. In people with IBS, those sensations can be amplified once you become aware of them and are difficult to turn off—not exactly opportune when you are trying to get to work. Instead, you're stuck with constant abdominal pain and urges to go to the bathroom. In this instance, the second brain, your gut's ENS, is taking over, and the big brain in your head (the CNS) is closely paying attention (perhaps way too much attention) to every signal coming through the pathway. If you are a "gut responder," you may find yourself being hit with GI symptoms in response to many of your day-to-day stressors. Research shows us that this is due in part to abnormalities in one's physiological stress response. Don't worry, *this can be changed*!

When you know your stress triggers (e.g., work deadlines, being overcommitted, travel) and you have tools to help mitigate the stress, GI-related symptoms can be improved. When you struggle with a gastrointestinal condition, knowing how to apply and use brain-gut-related therapies can be the key to stopping your GI symptoms in their tracks.

BRAIN-GUT BEHAVIORAL THERAPY FOR IBS 101

Rarely does medication work completely in the treatment of IBS, and everyone's experience is unique. Given the intertwined roles of the brain and the gut, behavioral therapies have emerged as an ideal way to treat symptoms that arise via this complicated pathway. As you step out of your medical provider's office and begin to think about what to do next, here are some of the science-backed and proven GI behavioral therapies that might pleasantly surprise you. The therapies summarized in Table 3 teach skills that can alleviate abdominal pain as well as other troubling symptoms like cramping, nausea, bloating, diarrhea, constipation, and other intestinal discomforts that drive IBS. In the coming chapters, we will teach you techniques from each type of therapy to fill your toolbox and improve your symptoms, with the goal of ultimately giving you the quality of life that you deserve.

Mind Your Gut

TABLE 3. TYPES OF BRAIN-GUT
BEHAVIORAL THERAPIES

	Underlying philosophy	Brain-gut benefit	Key skills
IBS self-management	The more you know about how your lifestyle affects your IBS, the better you can take charge of your health. Become a highly confident IBS self-management all-star!	Knowing that you have various options to address your IBS offers hope. Awareness of ways you can reduce IBS symptoms can improve your overall quality of life.	Create healthy habits for your nutrition, sleep, stress, self-care, mind-body interventions, exercise, and more.
Cognitive behavioral therapy (CBT)	Your outlook— on IBS and the world around you—affects the way you feel, how you behave, and how you manage IBS.	Addresses stress, negative emotions, thought processes, avoidance behaviors, and co-occurring depression and anxiety, all of which influence the way your brain and gut behave.	Unlearn the negative thought and behavior patterns that have developed due to your GI symptoms and stress. Techniques include cognitive restructuring, increasing cognitive flexibility, relaxation training, and more.

Gut-directed hypnotherapy	Achieving greater focus and awareness in a relaxed state may help you become more open to changing your experience with IBS.	Works on the brain-gut axis to address the effects of physical and emotional stress, negative and unhelpful thought patterns, and somatic symptoms common in IBS.	Learn how to deeply relax your body. Techniques (e.g., passive muscle relaxation and autogenous training) produce sensations of relaxation such as heaviness and warmth to normalize and restore brain-gut function.
Mindfulness-based stress reduction	Being grounded in the present moment, despite discomforts or pain, can help you recognize that suffering can lessen or pass.	Reduces suffering by decreasing awareness of your symptoms or improving how you manage them if they happen.	Engage in a regular practice of emotional and physical relaxation skills to ground yourself in times of stress.

MENTAL HEALTH MATTERS

Living life with irritable bowel syndrome is, well, irritating. Many patients say things like "If my IBS is behaving, my mood is good, and I can enjoy my life. If I'm having symptoms, they impact my mood and make me more likely to be anxious, on edge, and frustrated." Often those that do best with behavioral strategies recognize that IBS flare-ups affect their mood. Fortunately, as you will see in this book, especially in Chapters 2, 3, and 4, there are many behavioral strategies to lessen anxiety and stress that you can apply wherever you encounter your symptoms (e.g., at home, at work, in your car, on public transportation . . .). This book will provide you with many tactics for dealing with the common mood symptoms that are driven by your relationship with your digestive tract. As you learn to utilize effective tools, gone will be the times when your whole day is run—and ruined—by your IBS.

However, if you suffer from severe anxiety, depression, or post-traumatic stress, this book is not a substitute for mental health treatment that may be critical. IBS-specific behavioral interventions will not be as effective. It is important to get those conditions under control with the help of a licensed mental health provider. If you aren't sure where to turn for that kind of support, use the Resources in the back of this book as a starting point.

HOW FOOD MAY CAUSE GI DISTRESS IN IBS

Stress is one common denominator in IBS. The other is diet. Eating-related digestive distress occurs in upward of 80 percent of IBS patients.

To understand how certain foods, or even just the process of eating, can aggravate IBS, it's first important to understand some basics about the GI-tract anatomy. The digestive system's function is to transform the food you eat into energy for your body. The GI tract includes the mouth, esophagus, stomach, small intestine, and large intestine, or colon. Digestion starts in the mouth with chewing. Your teeth break up food, increasing its surface area, and allow the enzymes in your saliva to start the process of digestion. Chewing adequately is important for better digestion of your food. Here's a friendly reminder for everyone, particularly those with a GI condition: whenever you eat, relax, go slowly, and chew your foods well!

Chewed foods travel down the esophagus and into the stomach. The stomach produces acid and enzymes to digest foods further before the remnants enter the small intestine. The small intestine releases additional enzymes, along with enzymes from the pancreas and bile from the liver (stored in the gallbladder), to digest food into absorbable components. From the small intestine, nutrients are actively transported into the bloodstream to nourish the body. Meanwhile, undigested food (mostly fiber) travels to the colon. The main roles of the colon are to provide residence to important gut microbes that further break down foods and create important vitamins, to help the body absorb water, and to eliminate the end products of digestion.

There are several drivers of how food can trigger GI symptoms in IBS, and this area of study is a relatively new and rapidly expanding field. Food can influence a variety of physiologic factors that lead to IBS symptoms, such as changing intestinal motility (speeding it up or slowing it down), increasing visceral sensation (lowering the threshold to pain), making brain-gut interactions more pronounced, unfavorably changing the gut microbiome (reducing the variety of gut microbes or promoting the growth of potentially pathogenic microbes), increasing intestinal permeability (allowing microbes and their metabolites that normally stay within the colon to travel through the gut lining into other parts of the body), and activating the immune system, to name a few.

SOMETIMES IT'S THE WAY THE GUT MOVES, NOT THE SPECIFIC FOOD YOU EAT

While many people with IBS get focused on *what* they are eating, other eating-related factors (outside of specific foods) may contribute to symptoms. For example, do you frequently need to make a run for the bathroom right after you eat? The body has a physiological response called the gastrocolic reflex, which controls the motility of the lower-GI tract following a meal. In people with IBS, there tends to be a stronger colonic response to the gastrocolic reflex. That can lead to a strong urge to use the bathroom following a meal. Further, the more pronounced the colonic contractions, the more you may feel abdominal pain and the more sensitive you may be to abdominal distention and gas in the intestine. The act of eating, smelling, and even just seeing food can stimulate the gastrocolic reflex. (This is one reason why IBS symptoms rarely occur at night: people are not eating or smelling food when sleeping.)

Another important regulator of the small intestine is the migrating motor complex (MMC). Normally, the muscles in the stomach and small intestine move food through the intestine in a synchronized fashion; these series of contractions are called peristalsis. The upper digestive tract also undergoes a cyclic pattern of contractions known as the MMC. There are four phases of the MMC. Phase I is a quiet period with virtually no contractions. Phase II provides intermittent and irregular low-amplitude contractions. Phase III, known as the cleansing wave, provides quick bursts of high-amplitude contractions that essentially clean out the small intestine, moving food, secretions, and microbes. Phase IV provides a swift transition period back to the stillness of Phase I. The MMC-Phase III, or the cleansing wave, only occurs when food is *not* present in the gut—that is, during the fasting state, or about every 90 to 120 minutes in people with normal cleansing wave function. In individuals with altered intestinal motility, such as those with IBS, the cleansing waves occur less often.

If you are someone who tends to snack all day rather than eating at regular mealtimes, this could be throwing your MMC out of whack. Again, it's when you are *not* eating that your intestine will initiate the important MMC-Phase III that helps clear out the small intestine and get it ready for food again. Allowing some downtime is important; otherwise, your small intestine can become a petri dish, permitting microbes and food to interact and ferment, which may increase trapped gas and result in IBS symptoms. You want your small intestine to have the time to initiate a cleansing wave several times during the day. Eating three distinct meals and a snack versus grazing all day will better accommodate these important cleansing waves. Of course, that said, avoiding eating when hungry or trying to go as long as you can without eating is never the goal, as this pattern moves you away from tuning in to your body and honoring hunger signals. Always listen to your body!

FOOD-RELATED REACTIONS: WHAT'S THE DIFFERENCE?

Sometimes the body reacts negatively to a consumed food. In general, there are three types of food-related reactions: allergic, autoimmune, and intolerance. Table 4 offers a brief overview of the more common food-related reactions, the mechanisms that drive them, examples of potential diagnoses, and symptoms.

TABLE 4. FOOD-RELATED REACTIONS: ALLERGY, AUTOIMMUNE, AND INTOLERANCE

Food reaction	What drives the reaction?	Examples of clinical diagnoses	Symptoms
Allergy	IgE reactions, non-IgE reactions, occasional IgE reactions	True food allergy, FPIES, eosinophilic esophagitis	Respiratory, GI, cardiovascular, skin (dermatitis, hives), in severe cases multisystem anaphylaxis

Autoimmune	Innate and adaptive immune system	Celiac disease	GI symptoms, fatigue, low iron, osteoporosis, low B12, low folate, low zinc, weight loss or gain
Food intolerance	Disorder of digestive or absorptive process in small intestine, toxic or pharmacologic reactions	Lactose intolerance, sucrose/starch intolerance, IBS, FODMAP intolerance, histamine, A1 beta-casein intolerance	GI: uptick in intestinal gas, bloating, constipation or diarrhea, abdominal pain Other: hives, low blood pressure, headaches, abdominal pain

IgE: immunoglobulin E; FPIES: food protein–induced enterocolitis syndrome; FODMAP: fermentable oligosaccharides, disaccharides, monosaccharides, and polyols

"DO I HAVE A FOOD ALLERGY?"

A true food allergy certainly can occur in people with IBS; in fact, food allergies are on the rise, affecting about 11 percent of American adults. But food intolerance–based reactions in IBS (see page 29) are much more typical.

A food allergy reaction is an abnormal immune response to a food protein. Most allergic reactions occur as an immunoglobulin E (IgE) reaction. IgE is an antibody created by the immune system during the allergic response.

The most common IgE-mediated food allergies are triggered by nine foods: peanuts, tree nuts, milk, eggs, wheat, soy, fish, shellfish, and sesame seeds. Food allergic reactions can involve the skin, mouth, eyes, lungs, heart, gut, and even brain. They can be mild or severe, even life-threatening. Anaphylaxis occurs quickly after exposure to the allergen. Its symptoms include shortness of breath, nausea, vomiting, hives, swelling of lips and tongue, low blood pressure, wheezing, fainting, and cardiac arrest. Anaphylaxis involves the whole body and requires immediate medical attention (call 911). If you are at risk for anaphylaxis, your allergist will prescribe a self-injectable epinephrine pen and instructions on how to use it. Epinephrine relaxes the muscles in the airway to make breathing easier and helps maintain blood pressure. Diagnosis of food allergies is undertaken with the guidance of an allergist, who will take a detailed medical and symptom history and may recommend skin or blood tests to help determine if you have an allergy. Allergy tests offer some guidance about the presence of food allergies, but they do not confirm with 100 percent certainty that a food allergy exists. An oral food challenge is often used to confirm a food allergy after blood or skin tests have been completed.

FOOD INTOLERANCES: THE MOST LIKELY IBS CULPRITS

Food intolerances often contribute to IBS symptoms. They are extremely common, occurring in about one in five people globally. Food intolerances are not allergies; they are assorted reactions prompting digestive symptoms such as gas, bloating, abdominal cramping, and diarrhea or constipation. And unlike food allergies, intolerances are not life-threatening. Of course, even though a food-related reaction may not be deadly, living with it can be very disruptive to your daily life.

Food intolerance can occur due to osmotic effects (when a food pulls water into the gut and stretches it), fermentative effects (when gut microbes consume poorly digested foods, creating copious gas), mechanical effects (when large, insoluble fiber components, such as wheat bran, irritate the lining of the gut, stimulating mucus and water secretion), or pharmacologic effects (when food components prompt hives or diarrhea). Let's take a look at some of the common food intolerances in people with IBS.

Enzyme Deficiencies

Food intolerance may also occur due to a lack of certain digestive enzymes, such as those needed to digest the sugar lactose, found in some dairy products. In lactose intolerance, the body doesn't produce enough of the intestinal digestive enzyme lactase, resulting in poor digestion of lactose—the milk sugar found in cow, goat, and sheep milk—and leading to digestive distress. When the undigested lactose arrives in the colon, it pulls water into the gut and is fermented by gut microbes, creating gas. The aftermath is diarrhea and cramping. No fun!

Similarly, if your body doesn't make enough of the enzyme sucrase-isomaltase, you may experience symptoms akin to lactose intolerance. Without adequate levels of this enzyme, sucrose (found in table sugar, pastries, and some fruits and vegetables) and sometimes starch (found in potatoes, pasta, bread) are not well digested and are subsequently fermented by microbiota in the colon. While sucrase-isomaltase deficiency (SID) was once thought to be rare and diagnosed primarily in children, recent research has found that certain genetic alterations resulting in a reduction in the enzyme complex may be present in some adults with IBS, perhaps occurring in one out of ten people with IBS-D.

FODMAP Intolerance

Do onions and garlic give your gut trouble? Or maybe you've noticed that your symptoms get worse after eating stone fruits? Certain foods composed of small-chain sugars and fibers, collectively known as FODMAP carbohydrates, are major offenders in triggering digestive distress in IBS. "FODMAP" is an acronym for "fermentable oligosaccharides, disaccharides, monosaccharides, and polyols." (Say that five times fast!) While not all FODMAPs require specific enzymes for digestion and absorption, they tend to be poorly absorbed, particularly when consumed in larger amounts. And remember that the *F* stands for "fermentable," which means it creates gas. In IBS, FODMAP intolerance is common. In fact, about 50 to 80 percent of those with IBS will experience symptom relief with a low-FODMAP diet. Currently, a low-FODMAP diet has the most scientific evidence of all diets to back its use for IBS. For a breakdown of the foods rich in the various FODMAP carbohydrates, see Table 5.

TABLE 5. FODMAP SUBTYPES AND EXAMPLES OF THE MOST COMMON FOOD SOURCES

Subtype	Specific substances	Common food sources
Oligosaccharides	Water-soluble fibers, namely fructans and galacto-oligosaccharides (GOS)	Wheat, onion, garlic, legumes, barley, rye, watermelon, chicory root extract, asparagus, artichokes, hummus, kidney beans, soybeans, cashew and pistachio nuts, chamomile and fennel herbal tea, carob
Disaccharides (two-chain sugars)	Lactose	Milk, ice cream, yogurt, sour cream, ricotta, or cottage cheese made from cow, sheep, or goat milk

Monosaccharides (one-chain sugars)	Fructose (when present in excess of glucose in a food)	Apples, cherries, pears, mango, asparagus, watermelon, honey, agave nectar, rum
Polyols	Also known as sugar alcohols, including mannitol, sorbitol, isomalt, xylitol, maltitol	Stone fruits, such as cherries, plums, peaches, nectarines; blackberries; sorbitol-, xylitol-, or mannitol-based sugar-free gum and mints; cauliflower, most mushrooms

FODMAP-containing foods are not unhealthy or "bad." In fact, several are healthy and nourishing. But in many people with IBS, FODMAPs trigger gut symptoms (see Figure 2). How do FODMAPs cause GI distress?

1. Well, for starters, FODMAP carbohydrates are osmotically active, meaning they pull water into the small intestine, stretching the intestinal wall, which can contribute to pain, cramping, and bloating.

2. Further, the poorly digested FODMAPs arrive in the colon intact, becoming fast food for the trillions of microbes that reside there.

3. When the microbes feed off the FODMAPs, this act of fermentation creates gas and short-chain fatty acids (SCFAs). Although SCFAs can act as nourishing fuel for the cells of the colon, they also can speed up the colon's motility.

4. The extra water and gas in the gut stretch it farther, contributing to bloating and cramping in a person with a sensitive stomach.

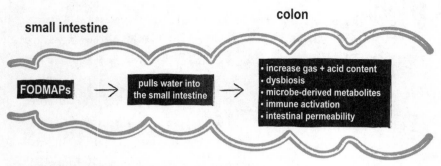

Figure 2. FODMAPs and GI Symptoms in IBS

5. Bacterial toxins may be produced that can trigger pain
    in the gut. New research has shown that fermentation of
    FODMAPs in some people can lead to growth of certain
    microbes that contain a bacterial toxin called lipopoly-
    saccharide. This scenario is associated with increased
    "leakiness of the gut" and with triggering mast cells
    (immune cells in the gut) to release inflammatory chem-
    icals that appear to generate pain.

Precisely how FODMAPs trigger symptoms in IBS is not yet
fully understood, but it appears to be a complex interaction between
our gut microbes, the foods we eat, and our immune systems. What
we do know is that reducing FODMAPs can be helpful for symptom
management in many people living with IBS. We'll dive deep into
how to get started on a low-FODMAP diet in Chapters 5 and 6.

GUT GAME CHANGER: LEAKY GUT *SYNDROME?*

Everyone's gut has some level of permeability (aka leakiness), which is normal. But excessive permeability (referred
to as leaky gut or increased intestinal permeability) is associated with some GI conditions, such as IBS and inflammatory

bowel disease. Some emerging science suggests that a low-FODMAP diet and/or supplementing with glutamine (an amino acid that fuels the gut) may help reduce leakiness in certain people with IBS.

That said, there is no scientific evidence for a condition called leaky gut *syndrome*. The word "syndrome" suggests it is a diagnosis on its own with potential treatment modalities. But no science-based therapies exist to treat so-called leaky gut syndrome. Be wary of health-care providers that state they treat this concocted condition.

Gluten Intolerance

You've probably heard the buzz about going gluten-free, or you've seen gluten-free food products at the supermarket and wondered if you should eliminate it from your diet. Gluten is a protein contained in the grains wheat, barley, and rye, which are ingredients in many foods, from pasta, bread, and baked goods to less obvious ones like soy sauce and some candies. Gluten is a known trigger in celiac disease (CD), an autoimmune condition in which gluten is downright toxic. In CD, gluten causes inflammation and flattening of the absorptive lining of the small intestine.

When it comes to IBS, interestingly, a gluten-free diet has been shown to reduce digestive symptoms. However, most studies that examine the role of gluten in IBS have uncovered that the benefit of a gluten-free diet in symptom reduction is a result of the reduction of FODMAP carbohydrate sources (fructans) that are also found in the gluten-containing grains. (We'll go into FODMAPs further in Chapters 5 and 6.) There may be a subset of people with IBS that do, in fact, experience true gluten intolerance, but based on the science to date, a food intolerance specific to the protein gluten appears to be a less common occurrence in IBS. A dietitian with expertise in GI conditions can provide guidance to determine if you are sensitive to either FODMAPs or gluten (or both) by administering specific food challenges and conducting symptom profiling.

A1 Beta-Casein Intolerance

Another instigator of digestive symptoms is an intolerance to A1 beta-casein, one of the main proteins in cow's milk (making up about 30 percent of the protein content). Beta-casein in cow's milk can have two forms, A1 and A2. While some cows produce solely A2 beta-casein, commercial milk production tends to pool all milks together; therefore, most commercial milk products contain both forms. Studies have shown that, for people with lactose intolerance, switching to a milk product with only A2 beta-casein resulted in a reduction of digestive complaints compared to consuming A1 beta-casein. Interestingly, sheep and goats produce only A2 beta-casein, which may explain why some individuals tolerate those forms of milk better.

Histamine Intolerance

Histamine intolerance is yet another potential food intolerance that can lead to digestive symptoms. Histamine, naturally found in some foods, is a nitrogen compound produced in part by living organisms such as gut microbes. The intolerance results from a decline in diamine oxidase (DAO), an enzyme produced in the small intestine that helps the body degrade dietary histamine. This can happen when there is intestinal inflammation—in conditions like IBS, celiac disease, inflammatory bowel disease, small intestinal bacterial overgrowth (SIBO), and others.

An example of histamine overload documented in the scientific literature is scombroid fish poisoning, or histamine fish poisoning, a syndrome that resembles an allergic reaction. It can happen after eating spoiled fish or fish that contains high levels of histamine.

Histamine-rich foods have been identified as food triggers in IBS patients. In one study of nearly two hundred IBS patients, 58 percent identified histamine-rich foods as culprits in GI symptoms. Histamine is in wine, beer, cured meats, aged cheese, some canned fish, some fruits, and vegetables. Interestingly, spinach has been shown to be a high-histamine vegetable, in part due to the microbes naturally living on the leaves, which produce histamine. If you and your GI dietitian or other health provider suspect that histamine is a trigger for your symptoms, a short-term trial of a modified-histamine diet may be warranted. Just bear in mind that the diet has not been adequately studied in a research setting, and understanding of how to apply a low-histamine diet is limited.

Intolerance to Fatty Foods

Everyone loves french fries, but our gut doesn't always love them back. Another food intolerance reaction can occur with the overconsumption of fatty foods. Fat may contribute to digestive distress in IBS because it can reduce small intestinal motility, resulting in trapped gas and abdominal bloating. Further, fat can exacerbate the gastrocolic reflex. As we discussed earlier, the gastrocolic response typically occurs after eating a meal. If you find that eating fatty foods results in an urgent trip to the bathroom, it may be due to an exaggeration in this reflex. Some common fatty-food triggers include fried foods (e.g., french fries, doughnuts, fried fish platters), creamy soups, and rich desserts.

Intolerance to Insoluble Fiber

Too much insoluble fiber, found in the skins of fruits and veggies as well as in wheat bran, might also trigger your IBS symptoms.

Wheat bran specifically has been shown in scientific studies to exacerbate IBS—and it's found in many whole-grain wheat breads, crackers, cereals, and bran muffins. The bran itself can irritate the colonic mucosa and trigger secretion of mucus and water.

Adjusting your intake of fat and insoluble fiber, under the guidance of a GI dietitian, can help reduce your digestive symptoms. There is no need, however, to eat an extremely low-fat diet or to eliminate all insoluble fiber foods to manage gut symptoms in IBS. We find that a few tweaks can be enough. For example, an easy way to reduce insoluble fiber could be to switch to multi-grain bread instead of 100 percent whole wheat, or to spread your fat intake throughout the day instead of eating a very rich meal at one sitting.

DIETS FOR IBS

There are three dietary approaches most often used to counter IBS: "traditional," also known as the National Institute for Health and Care Excellence (NICE) IBS diet (from the United Kingdom), which consists of lifestyle and nutritional changes; a gluten-free diet; and the low-FODMAP diet. These are summarized in Table 6. Again, the low-FODMAP diet has the strongest science to support its use and appears to be the most likely to reduce IBS symptoms. But continue to watch this space, as research looking at a Mediterranean diet is of interest in IBS and is now being explored in the research setting. It shows some promising benefits for GI and psychological symptoms. A Mediterranean diet is rich in plant foods, including a variety of fruits, vegetables, and legumes, as well as extra-vrigin olive oil, fish, nuts, and some dairy and poultry too.

TABLE 6. DIETS COMMONLY APPLIED FOR
IBS SYMPTOM MANAGEMENT

Low-FODMAP diet	Three-phase nutritional approach that includes elimination phase (high-FODMAP foods are removed), reintroduction phase (FODMAPs are added back systematically to find food triggers), and personalization phase (tolerated FODMAP foods are added back to the diet)
National Institute for Health and Care Excellence IBS diet	Diet and lifestyle changes that include eating three meals per day and not missing meals; reducing alcohol, caffeine, spicy foods; increasing fluids; minimizing fat; and altering fiber intake (adding soluble fiber)
Gluten-free (GF) diet (The benefit of a GF diet appears to be due to a reduction of co-occurring FODMAPs)	All gluten sources are eliminated from the diet; gluten is a protein found in wheat, barley, and rye

Given that eating food is both an essential part of life and a potential source of IBS distress, food-related worry, anxiety, and avoidance are common. In fact, in a 2022 study of 955 patients with IBS, 54 percent reported that they frequently avoided food because of IBS. The avoidance of food is often related to the anxiety of looming GI symptoms after a meal (e.g., "If I don't eat, I might not have these terrible symptoms"). As you read through this book, you'll find strategies for making positive changes to your nutrition and your mind; the two go hand in hand in managing your IBS symptoms. You will be guided in the very latest science in nutrition and the low-FODMAP diet, as well as in other dietary adaptations to explore.

When possible, consult with a GI-expert dietitian to help navigate changes to your diet. They can help you tease out your individual food triggers—which may be uncommon—and maximize your nutrition without overly restricting foods. The goal of any dietary approach to IBS is to enjoy the most liberal, nourishing, and delicious diet possible while successfully managing symptoms so that you can enjoy a full life!

GUT GAME CHANGER:
INTEGRATED MEDICAL CENTERS

Integrated medical centers that focus on IBS typically combine the forces of expert dietitians, gastroenterologists, and psychologists (the Dream Team model). Professionals in these fields know the power of working together! Often the patients we work with had no idea this type of integrative approach was available. You are not alone, and we have strategies to decrease that food- and gut-related worry.

IT'S PERSONAL: INDIVIDUALIZING THE BEST SCIENCE-BASED APPROACH FOR *YOU*

Because IBS presents in diverse ways and is often triggered by different things, a personalized approach will offer the best outcome. That means *you* are at the center: understanding your triggers, symptoms, history, values, and motivations is what is most important. IBS management is not one-size-fits-all, so we will provide you with a variety of science-proven treatments to help you feel your best. These range from the art of deep breathing to healing recipes that will soothe your tummy when it needs it most. We've also designed our recipes to make your taste buds sing, because delicious food can be a beautiful aspect of life, and maybe you've been missing it for a while.

WHEN FLARE-UPS STRIKE

It's no secret, IBS flares can sneak up on us. In her clinical practice, Kate often uses the analogy that living with IBS is like walking on a balance beam. You require a bit more structure and good form to avoid falling, compared with someone without IBS, whose feet are firmly on the ground. You can stay in line and stay on the beam with some careful adjustments, but certain triggers may tip you off the beam. The fall represents a flare.

While IBS is a chronic condition and symptoms can settle and flare in an unpredictable sequence, sometimes we receive subtle messages from our body that gut symptoms are going a bit south. If you can preemptively make some changes by using your IBS toolkit, you can often abort a full-on flare. For example, in those with constipation-predominant IBS, tuning into elimination patterns that may have slowed a bit by taking an extra walk, revisiting your laxative medications, or whipping up a Clean-Sweep Take-2 Smoothie (recipe on page 290) might just be your free pass from an IBS flare. In IBS-D, when bloating and diarrhea amp up, a slight reduction in FODMAPs for a day or two may be just enough to quell your gut and avoid a major uptick in symptoms. At other times, you may find that stress is a bigger factor, and engaging in key de-stress measures such as pulling back on extra commitments, engaging in your practice of diaphragmatic breathing (page 57), or adding a yoga class may be more of what you need for a gut reset.

When a flare strikes, give yourself some grace. It's not your fault. Allow a fall from the beam to be a learning moment for you to identify what may have led to the fall. You might have been enjoying a few more cocktails than usual, or maybe you didn't notice that you hadn't had a cleansing bowel movement for a week, or your stress level is over the top. When you see patterns emerging that tend to result in a flare, you can take note and dial back on your diet, ramp up on your laxative program, say no more frequently, or simply make more time to rest. Remember, the goal is not to strive for perfection with your sensitive gut but rather to achieve incremental gains and a better understanding of what works best for your body.

As you read through this book and make use of the various tools, fill out the Mind Your Gut My Essentials for Health List (page 317). It will be a great resource for you when a flare occurs. Look over the form and reengage in the tools that you found most useful to settle your gut.

In the meantime, here are a few well-tested IBS flare-management tips for you to try:

- A warm bath can help relax all the body's muscles, including those in the gut.
- Calm your mind and your digestive tract with a few minutes of diaphragmatic breathing (page 57) a couple of times throughout the day.
- Try a gentle abdominal "I love you" massage (page 112) to help move out any trapped gas.
- Sip on ginger tea, which can quell nausea and aid stomach emptying.
- Rest on your back with a heating pad over your tummy.
- Try enteric-coated peppermint, which helps relax the smooth muscles in your gut and has been shown to have direct antimicrobial and anti-inflammatory effects as well as to reduce IBS symptoms.
- Put on some coffeehouse music or spa music, light a candle, and let those environmental cues encourage you and your body to transition into a relaxed state.
- Deepen your relaxation response with the gut-directed relaxation interventions provided in Chapter 4.

It's time to think differently about living with IBS. The very good news is that research on IBS is experiencing a renaissance. More therapeutic options are being studied, and we now know how to manage the condition better than ever. In this book you will find chapters that focus on the gut and brain connection, others with a nutrition focus, and still others that weave together treatment options to target the stubborn symptoms that nag you most. Turn the page and start learning—it's time to feel better! We care about you and are glad to have you as part of the team.

CHAPTER 2

WHEN YOUR GUT AND BRAIN TALK TOO MUCH

Do you know what often leads to symptom flare-ups and worse IBS? It's *stress*. You may be surprised that stress can have such a deep physical impact, but it's true. Researchers have extensively studied the pathophysiology of IBS and have found that psychological stress (which can include chronic stress, adverse events in childhood, and trauma) is a leading factor. Emerging research from the University of California, Los Angeles, shows that adverse events in childhood happened at similar rates in women and men with IBS. Therefore, understanding the role of stress and how you can effectively manage it in the here and now is important for everyone with IBS.

Unfortunately, the stress of having IBS can itself fuel a vicious cycle. While it is normal to worry about persistent digestive symptoms, when the worry and anxiety become unrelenting, IBS typically gets worse. What is there to worry about? Well, we hear it all: feeling controlled by the unpredictability of your bowels; having to take time away from school, work, and family; dealing with mounting bills from doctor's appointments; navigating a medical odyssey— all the workups, procedures, medications, supplements. . . . The list goes on.

HOW DOES STRESS AFFECT IBS?

The effects of stress on your gut can be profound, and they range from affecting the cellular makeup of your intestines to how sensitive you are to pain. Stress can:

- **Disrupt the interactions between the brain and gut.** Stress affects the bidirectional pathway of the brain-gut axis. Stress can also result in overactivity or underactivity of the hypothalamic-pituitary-adrenal (HPA) axis and of the autonomic nervous, metabolic, and immune systems. Ultimately this affects different physiological functions of the gastrointestinal tract.
- **Increase intestinal permeability.** Greater intestinal permeability, or "leakiness" of the gut, allows potentially harmful toxins into the bloodstream and has been found to be a key factor in the severity of IBS complications and GI pain.
- **Alter the secretions and motility (movement) of the intestine** by slowing down or speeding up bowel transit, contractions, and movement through the GI system. This may cause pain as well as constipation, diarrhea, or both.
- **Contribute to increased visceral hypersensitivity,** which is experienced as bloating and abdominal pain and can worsen bowel urgency.
- **Reshape the gut's bacterial composition** via changes in the stress hormones. Interestingly, our gut microbes can

upregulate stress responses and increase the risk of depression. Stress-induced changes to our gut microbes can alter mood and eating behavior (by, for example, triggering cravings for highly palatable foods that are often processed or flavored with alluring combinations of sugar, carbohydrates, sodium, and fat). You will learn a lot more about these fascinating gut microbes in Chapter 8.

Much of the communication between the gut and the brain takes place without us actually being aware of it. However, regardless of what triggers your symptoms, the brain is ultimately responsible for generating the conscious perception of those pesky abdominal and bowel symptoms based on sensory input coming from your gut. As you learned, the mechanisms by which the brain and the gut function are controlled by the enteric nervous system (ENS), located in the walls of the digestive tract. The ENS is a built-in safety patrol for our body. It assesses our surroundings and works to keep the body in ready position to act if necessary. The sympathetic nervous system (best known for its role in helping our body respond to danger or stressful situations) helps us fight, flight, or freeze, while the parasympathetic nervous system responds to calm our body at the right time. The parasympathetic system is our internal relaxation response system and is vital in assisting with digesting.

Sometimes, based on the severity of the life stress you have experienced, your body may respond to day-to-day stress in a way that ramps up your gut and makes it more difficult to bounce back to the things you want and need to be doing. Thankfully, your body and mind are incredibly resilient and can be taught how to manage the stress response. Throughout this chapter, you will learn what to avoid when it comes to living well with IBS (see you later, snake oil!). Instead, we will teach you to recognize the GI stress cycle and will supply you with effective management strategies to mitigate stress and create healthy relaxation habits you will look forward to implementing every day.

VISCERAL HYPERSENSITIVITY: IT'S A MIND AND GUT PHENOMENON

In people living with IBS, some of the wiring between the brain and gut misfires. The result of this faulty wiring is one of the root causes of IBS: visceral hypersensitivity. This term refers to abnormal pain sensing in the GI tract that results from overstimulation of the stress response.

First things first: your pain is very *real*! There is nothing about the pain from gas, bloating, cramping, or spasming that is made up or "in your head." However, research shows that people with IBS feel normal gut sensations (i.e., the digestive process) that most people would not be aware of, and when you feel those sensations, they are more painful than what others without IBS would experience. The increased gut sensations often lead to increased stress and increased pain.

The good news is that certain GI-based behavioral therapies, such as cognitive behavioral therapy (CBT), mindfulness training, and hypnotherapy, can actually reduce the hypersensitive nature of the gut. In fact, it is hypothesized that gut-directed hypnotherapy decreases sensitivity to visceral sensations, which helps to normalize gut function over time. This means *you* can improve that faulty wiring!

Visceral hypersensitivity has a partner in crime in the form of visceral anxiety, which is a type of anxiety experienced by many people with IBS. Visceral anxiety happens when a GI sensation (such as a gurgle, spasm, or cramp) or situation (eating out with friends, commuting to work, going to a concert) triggers unhelpful thoughts or behaviors. These unhelpful responses can come in the form of heightened awareness of your GI sensations (sensitivity). This leads to paying so much attention (hypervigilance) to your GI sensations that you limit your focus and ability to do other things besides experiencing fear, worry, and avoidance. The use of strategies to confront fears and to stop avoiding situations that make you anxious can be learned through exposure therapy techniques: you learn through repeated exposure that the likelihood of the feared outcome is much lower than predicted and that you are capable of handling it. When you have the skills to notice that this type of anxiety is ramping up, you will be able to get ahead of your gut—and reduce the chance of worsened pain by utilizing more effective coping skills.

ANXIETY AND ANSWER SEEKING IN IBS

Anxiety lives in life's unknowns. We all experience some anxiety when we are thrown into an uncontrollable situation. When IBS enters the picture, we see people desperately doing everything they can to get better because of worry, fear, and debilitation. Two questionnaire-based studies illustrate the extent of this suffering. In the first study, people with IBS were willing to accept a 1 percent risk of sudden death from a hypothetical medication in return for a 99 percent chance of a cure for their IBS. In the second study, people with IBS were willing to give up 25 percent of their remaining life expectancy to be free of IBS symptoms.

Unfortunately, there are people out there who will sell you snake oil by taking advantage of anxiety related to your health. Whereas antidiarrheals, laxatives, pain relievers, probiotics, prebiotics, and other supplements work for some people with IBS, they aren't the golden ticket for all. If your doctor has recommended them and they provide the relief you have been looking for, by all means, continue to take them as prescribed! However, be cautious of interventions that produce minimal or short-term effects, or that cause anxiety about whether stopping use of the product could worsen your symptoms.

We've seen patients who aren't sure to what extent their regimen is working but are nonetheless fearful of stopping it. We offer two key considerations regarding whether you should stick to your treatment: Is your quality of life good? And are you living as close to symptom-free as possible? All too often, patients follow treatment plans that fail to provide those outcomes: Luckily you are in the right place to receive additional suggestions that go beyond what can be picked up over the counter or at the pharmacy. But first, we've outlined some potential problems to be aware of in your search for symptom relief.

Watch for Red Flags

We don't want you to get caught up in the false promises found in the world of IBS pseudoscience. Pseudoscience involves interventions that seem compelling for your health problem but can prey on your anxiety and take advantage of you and others who are suffering. One can easily Google "treatment for IBS" and quickly find a variety of people from helping professions offering options that fit the category of pseudoscience or snake oil. These interventions typically make claims that are not based in scientific evidence and lack the rigorous scrutiny that true evidence-based interventions undergo.

Before investing your time, hard-earned money, and hope on a treatment for your IBS, be on the lookout for these red flags:

- Bold claims ("the cure") relying on case examples without data
- A guarantee that the treatment will fix "the root cause" of your symptoms
- A lack of high-quality, scholarly research testing the intervention
- Questionable explanations for how the treatment actually works

Be Careful with Supplements

While supplements are often touted to be a "safe and natural" approach to IBS self-management, there can be a downside. If you take supplements in excess, or supplements that aren't right for your condition, the digestive system can become overwhelmed, which can lead to intolerance. For example, a well-intentioned person can begin taking magnesium (often touted to calm the gut and "nerves") and find that the dosage actually causes even more diarrhea than they were already struggling with! Yes, too much magnesium can, in fact, cause diarrhea. Supplements to boost fiber or provide prebiotics for "gut health" may contain inulin or chicory root—common IBS trigger ingredients. Taking too many supplements at one time can make it difficult to decipher what is helping and what is worsening your symptoms. Work with your health-care provider to weed out excess supplement use to limit the potential downside to your digestive tract.

This is not to say that all supplements are bad—we'll delve into them further, and in Chapters 8 and 9 (as well as in the Resources), we recommend several to consider as part of your treatment plan based on specific IBS symptoms. But it is critical to work with a licensed medical provider or registered dietitian who will regularly assess how you are responding to a supplement and make adjustments—or will recommend that you stop if you are not experiencing improvement. Be mindful of people making recommendations outside the scope of their practice or those who are not licensed by an accredited organization. For example, anyone can call themselves a "nutritionist." Look for a registered dietitian to work with.

Bottom line: Remember to always check with your health-care provider before trying a new supplement.

Avoid Colonics for "Detox"

If you have had a colonoscopy, you essentially underwent a colonic or colon cleansing beforehand. The prep for a colonoscopy is done under the instruction of a medical physician for the purposes of preparing your digestive tract for a medical procedure. However, some people may seek out a colonic for so-called detoxification under the misguided belief that it will improve their immune system, increase their energy, or remove toxins that they believe are causing GI distress. Currently, there is no evidence to support colonics in reaching these effects. It's critical to understand that a colonic can be harmful or even dangerous. Potential side effects may include bloating, cramping, spasming, diarrhea, nausea, and vomiting. (More GI symptoms!) Additional concerns include dehydration, infection, and changes in electrolyte balance, which could be dangerous for those with certain health conditions. As if that's not enough, due to the nature of the colonic procedure, during which large amounts of water and sometimes other substances (such as herbs or coffee) are flushed through a tube inserted into the rectum, there is also risk of rectal perforation or tearing. Say no to colonics!

GUT GAME CHANGER: BEWARE OF MAGIC-BULLET MARKETING

You may find that marketers use phrases like the following to try to reel you in and get you to buy their services or supplement:

- "Quick fix"
- "Miracle pill"
- "What your doctor isn't telling you"
- "Tackle the root cause of IBS"
- "Cure your gut"

When struggling with pain, it's normal to want a quick-and-easy treatment. We get it! Unfortunately, when it comes to IBS treatments that are science-based and truly work, it's about the long game.

BREAKING THE GI STRESS CYCLE

"Oh no, my stomach. It hurts. This is not good. I can't get to the bathroom right now. Sh*t, here we go again."

Situations that involve being in confined places and spaces, where you feel as though lack of access to a bathroom is a threat, may activate your GI stress response. If you have ever been in a classroom, boardroom, grocery store, shopping mall, car, boat, train, plane . . . and felt a twinge in your stomach followed by a flush of warmth, muscle tension, and then worry or panic, you have experienced the GI stress cycle. In the moments when you felt your stomach, you likely had anxious or panicky thoughts. This type of thinking jump-starts the alarm system in your brain, activating the sympathetic nervous system, which will cause your muscles to tense, your breathing to become shorter and shallower, and maybe some perspiration, all of which can worsen GI distress. The GI distress then impairs the thoughts about the stressful situation, and you find yourself stuck in the GI stress cycle, feeling helpless and at the mercy of your IBS.

If you have been here (and let's face it, even people without IBS can be affected by this type of stress cycle), we've got tremendous news! Remember the parasympathetic nervous system? That incredible built-in relaxation response can be activated by *you*, by your own responses and behaviors! In fact, the action of the parasympathetic nervous system is one of the reasons why a person won't die from a panic attack. It may feel like you could, but the parasympathetic nervous system kicks in and returns the bodily activation that happens in a panic attack to baseline.

The key to breaking the GI stress cycle is to meet it with a relaxation response when you feel it coming on. Relaxation strategies will decrease the sympathetic activation that floods the brain and body and worsens GI symptoms. Figure 3 illustrates the GI stress cycle and introduces what we call cycle breakers for living well with IBS. You will grow confident in using these science-backed strategies.

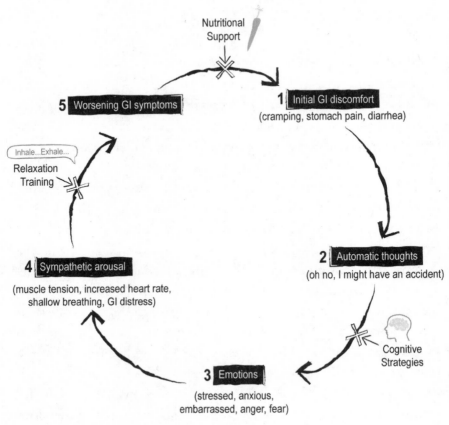

Figure 3. The GI Stress Cycle and Cycle Breakers

BRAIN BITE: A TRICK FOR PANIC ATTACKS

IBS symptoms may be especially problematic for people diagnosed with anxiety disorders that include panic disorder due to the revving of the sympathetic system that can occur during the GI stress cycle. Panic attacks are episodes of sudden and intense anxiety presenting as fear, repetitive worry, and doom, accompanied by physical symptoms of breathlessness, tightness in the chest, rapid heartbeat, nausea, sweating, dizziness, and at times a sensation that you might collapse or even die. It can feel as though the uncomfortable sensations of panic will last forever. If you are experiencing a panic attack, here's what to do:

- Begin to ground yourself in the present moment, and locate a clock.
- While looking at the clock, remind yourself that your body will naturally start to calm within about ten minutes.
- Focus on the clock, and tell yourself, "This will pass. I can focus on slowing down my breath. Inhale ... one, exhale ... two, inhale ... three, exhale ... four." Go all the way up to ten, then start again if needed.

We suggest working with a general mental health professional if panic attacks are affecting your day-to-day life.

READY, SET, RELAXATION RESPONSE

The strategies outlined later in the chapter involve cultivating a state of mind that may feel a bit different and requires practice, like learning a new language. Below, Dr. Riehl describes how she helps patients begin with small changes:

I often tell my patients that when learning stress management and relaxation interventions, change for the better will come with practice. The good news is that habits can be created in a fairly short period of time—but they do take time and repetition (research shows an average of sixty-six days). For example, early in the management of IBS, I begin by empowering the person with a strategy we were all born with: diaphragmatic breathing. We practice during the office session, and we discuss all the times that it will be most beneficial for them to practice the skill on their own—for example, when they experience bowel urgency, while attempting a bowel movement, after eating, before bed, while driving in the car, before taking an exam, to name a few. I remind them to practice when they find themselves in any of these scenarios before they return for their next appointment.

Several times, I have had someone return to that second session feeling frustrated and telling me that they attempted to use diaphragmatic breathing once or twice when they really needed relief, and "it didn't work." With compassion, I share this example: You would not walk out of your first French lesson and return to class a week later discouraged that you didn't become fluent in French over the week. That would be impossible! As with learning a foreign language, you do not become "fluent" in diaphragmatic breathing or other mind-body skills, like relaxation, without regular practice. So keep at it! Also, having various relaxation tools in your toolbox is helpful. You will identify, learn, and practice key strategies that you can engage to minimize IBS distress when you need it most. As you begin to reap the benefits of calming your nerves, it is likely that you will look forward to using these healthy habits.

You can use stress management techniques both reactively and proactively. Let's say you're in the car when, all of a sudden, you start experiencing cramps. But you are three miles from the next rest stop. An example of reactive stress management includes using diaphragmatic breathing to calm your body in response to the stressor. You can gain confidence by just knowing that how you respond in moments of discomfort might make a big difference in the outcome of a stressful situation.

An example of proactive stress management might be to plan to take a daily mindful moment (we'll teach you how) around lunchtime to check in with yourself emotionally. You are using strategies to manage daily stress before something "happens." A morning meditation practice, your daily physical exercise, diaphragmatic breathing after a meal to help with healthy digestion: these are a few examples of ways you can proactively utilize strategies that are good for your body and mind even if "nothing is happening."

CHECK IN WITH YOUR EMOTIONAL SIGNS

In moments of stress, it can be easy to get swept away in your thoughts. But behind your thinking is an emotion. If you don't take time to identify the emotion, it is harder to identify what coping strategy you may need. We'd like you to tune in to how you are feeling and use that to guide what happens next. Let's say you are running late one morning because your stomach was acting up and you had more bowel movements (BMs) than normal. Now you are rushing, skipping breakfast, and beginning to feel overwhelmed by the day before you are even out the door. It may seem counterintuitive, but this is a good time to take a pause. It doesn't take long. Ask yourself, "How am I really feeling right now?"

Maybe the answer is *I feel overwhelmed. I feel stressed. I feel frustrated.* Whatever you are feeling, recognize the power in identifying the emotions and the necessity of taking a few moments to calm yourself down before things escalate further. Often allowing yourself a little bit of time to observe the signs your mind and body are sending you is enough to shift the outcome of the stressful situation.

We know from research that feelings can have a big impact on pain. In fact, many studies show the importance of addressing negative emotions and stress due to their potential impact of causing, worsening, or prolonging pain conditions. We will introduce the use of a thought record in Chapter 3 as a tool that will help you identify not only the thoughts that you are thinking but the emotions that are present alongside them. The act of identifying the emotion and assessing the severity of that emotion is a powerful technique on its own. Sometimes you may think you are intensely experiencing an emotion, but then when you compare it to other times you felt that way, you may see that you have experienced it more strongly in the past—and survived! Table 7 lists emotions that you may experience in times of difficulty or stress—or even during positive events—and the bodily sensations that can go with them.

TABLE 7. EMOTIONS AND THE SENSATIONS THAT MAY ACCOMPANY THEM

Uncomfortable emotion	Sad	Scared	Angry	Embarrassed
Bodily sensations	Crying or tearing up, low energy, pressure in the chest	Shakiness, stomach discomfort, urge to avoid, freezing up or becoming tense	Muscle tension, urge to avoid, shakiness, stomach upset, feeling hot	Red in the face, nausea, stomach clenching, urge to avoid
Comfortable emotion	Playful/ excited	Confident	Loved	Happy
Bodily sensations	High energy, moving the body, engaged with others, laughter	Relaxed muscles, good energy, sound sleep, laughter	Calmness, peacefulness, desire to connect to others, warm body	Smiling, laughter, desire to connect physically, seeking out others

As you become more in tune with your emotions, you can establish a routine of healthy coping strategies to regulate your responses to them, which will ultimately help you regulate their effects on your gut.

FIVE STRATEGIES FOR CALM

The rest of the chapter discusses Dr. Riehl's five favorite strategies for calm. You can turn to these when you need a tummy time-out.

1. Diaphragmatic Breathing

When we asked our patients at the University of Michigan who were receiving brain-gut behavioral therapies what calming techniques they found most useful and would stick with after the conclusion of therapy, a whopping 91 percent said diaphragmatic breathing. It's free, easy, and ever-present. Diaphragmatic breathing, also referred to as belly breathing or relaxed breathing, offers several benefits for those with IBS. It is also beneficial for other GI concerns, such as heartburn associated with gastroesophageal reflux disease (GERD). By tempering the autonomic nervous system, it has a calming effect on the brain and on the cardiovascular, respiratory, and GI systems.

During times of stress or discomfort, our breathing tends to naturally become short, shallow, and even constrictive. (Have you ever had to remind yourself to breathe?) The diaphragm is a muscle that sits under the lungs. If you run your hands under your ribs, you will get an idea of where it is located. The activation of the diaphragm through deep breathing allows for a gentle massage of the internal organs. This remarkable technique can aid with abdominal pain or cramping, bowel urgency, bloating, constipation, and, as mentioned previously, uncomfortable reflux symptoms. Knowing how to use diaphragmatic breathing will provide you with an on-the-spot coping strategy to activate your body's relaxation response whenever you need it. It's a truly wondrous intervention!

> ## GUT GAME CHANGER:
> ## HELP FOR HEARTBURN
>
> Hypersensitivity, visceral anxiety, and stress can exacerbate upper-GI conditions, such as heartburn. Diaphragmatic breathing can ease heartburn and reflux that come on after eating by increasing the difference in pressure between the lower esophageal sphincter and the stomach.

If you experience diarrhea and bowel urgency, diaphragmatic breathing can assist in those moments of panic, such as when you are stuck in traffic or struck with the urge to go in public and there's not a bathroom in sight. Panic and anxiety will only worsen urgency, as we learned with the GI stress cycle. Purposefully shifting to slow, diaphragmatic breathing will provide you with a distraction from both the physical and the emotional discomfort that happen with urgency. Stress speeds up intestinal motility (how fast or slow stool moves through the gut), while slowed breathing can calm and slow down the digestive tract. Bonus: You are also getting a nice internal massage through the movement of the diaphragm.

Diaphragmatic breathing is also helpful if you are constipated. When someone is constipated, they may experience panic, frustration, and stress related to the desire or urge to have a bowel movement, only to experience the dread of an incomplete BM. These emotions, coupled with straining to defecate, can really wreak havoc on the body and mind. Further, physical stress and tension also affect intestinal motility.

Here's how to poop effectively while applying diaphragmatic breathing. First, engage the proper pooping position needed for a healthy bowel movement. Rest your feet on a low stand (such as the Squatty Potty—which, believe it or not, is *not* IBS snake oil!). This position is designed to keep your knees above your hips. Now, with a straight spine, lean slightly forward, to about a thirty-five-degree angle. (Learn more about the proper pooping position in the Resources section.)

Next, while maintaining this position, begin diaphragmatic breathing, which can soothe, relax, and massage your colon and other digestive organs while engaging the pelvic floor muscles. This helps to move stool out for an easier and more complete bowel movement.

Becoming comfortable with a daily diaphragmatic breathing practice is a great nonpharmaceutical option for improving your overall digestive symptoms and well-being.

Let's Practice Diaphragmatic Breathing

To begin, place one hand on your belly and one hand on your chest. Your hands will serve as a guide while you become comfortable with the practice. Your top hand should remain steady while your bottom hand will gently rise and fall with your breath. As you slowly breathe in, your lungs will fill completely, and the diaphragm will contract. As you slowly breathe out, your lungs push out the air and the diaphragm returns to its natural dome-like shape.

Breathe in through your nose for a count of four seconds. Pause for one or two seconds, and then exhale through your mouth for a count of six seconds. This count is just a guide and can be modified based on your comfort. The goal is for your exhale to be slightly longer than your inhale.

Often it will take practice for this to feel comfortable, as most people by nature are chest breathers. Begin with sessions of about ten breaths, and practice one to three times a day. As diaphragmatic breathing becomes more comfortable, you can use it without much thought in any situation, whether for on-demand symptom management, stress management, or to give yourself a moment of peace. See the Resources section for a link and a QR code for a video demonstration with Dr. Riehl.

2. The Mindful Minute

As we go through our day, our activity level, thoughts, needs, and pressures all increase. Without intentional stress management, all those stressors can take an emotional and physical toll. Maybe you have experienced that 2:00 p.m. slump when you find yourself distracted, daydreaming, or trying to multitask without making much progress. These are signals that your body and brain need a break (and maybe a nutritious meal or snack too). Your mind may say that you don't have time for a break. However, you aren't working at your full potential anyway, so you don't have much to lose.

Mindfulness involves paying attention in a focused way to the present moment, without judgment. The moment may be one of joy, one of sadness, or likely something in between. It isn't your job to change the situation at that moment; just observe it. Mindfulness is rooted in Buddhist meditation but has also become a well-researched intervention to reduce stress, cope with pain, boost the immune system, manage emotions, improve connection to others, and more.

Enter the mindful minute. This is a purposeful opportunity to check in with yourself, decrease physical and emotional stress, and return to your day feeling more focused, energized, and motivated. The power of the mindful minute lies in the fact that one of the most reliable and present things in life is your breath. You can't go back in time and breathe, and you can't breathe for the future. You can only do it now. Therefore, focusing on your breath grounds you in the present moment and assists with how you will cope with what comes next.

Let's Practice the Mindful Minute

Find a comfortable seated position. Set a timer for one minute; set the alarm to a low volume or a vibration for a less jarring conclusion to your practice. Close your eyes, and begin to focus on the rhythm of your breath, perhaps paying attention to your in-breath and out-breath for about two cycles. Start your timer, and continue to focus attention on your breath. Notice the sensation of your inhalation through your nose and the sound of your exhalation through your mouth. If a thought comes into your awareness, observe it, and then refocus on your breathing. Continue until your timer goes off. When you are ready, open your eyes and return to your day.

Feel free to lengthen your practice beyond one minute. You may also find great benefit in taking a brief mindful moment with your eyes open when in the presence of a beautiful spot in nature, or when you intentionally want to capture the moment with all your available senses. Recognize that these shorter interventions are meant to be easily implemented and used frequently.

3. Meditation

The practice of meditation can take many different forms. Often people feel that it is too hard to begin a meditation practice with a traditional "sit and clear your mind" exercise. Many people with IBS who live busy and productive lives have a hard time "not thinking of anything." Meditation is often misconstrued as a rigid practice, but there are various ways to do it. The first step is showing a willingness to experiment to discover what you enjoy and find helpful. Start out small and take baby steps toward the form of meditation that works for you. Beginners might find that having someone guide them through a practice is helpful. Nowadays there are tons of apps, websites, online programs, and in-person meditation studios where you can find a guide or program. See the Resources for suggestions to get you started.

Before you begin your meditation practice, you will want to set yourself up for success by learning a little about the different ways you can meditate. Depending on the type of meditation, the setup will differ slightly. However, the goal of using meditation to enhance your health transcends the various postures. You are encouraged to modify any practice in a way that feels right for your body. As your practice develops, you might find that when you are feeling a certain way, you turn to a certain type of meditation. For example, if you are worried about something and have started to get a stomachache in anticipation, shifting to a seated meditation practice to bring focus and attention back to the present moment may help decrease the effects of your worry on your IBS. Here's a rundown of some typical meditation postures.

Seated meditation: When doing a seated practice, think about a space where you will be able to focus and bring awareness to yourself. Often, sitting is thought to be an ideal position as it allows for just the right balance between a relaxed body and a focused mind. You may choose to sit on a chair with your feet planted on the ground. You can place your bum in the middle of the chair with a pillow or blanket supporting your lower back so that you aren't slumping forward or backward. The main goals are to have a relaxed, straight back, with head and neck in line with your spine, and arms resting in your lap, on your legs, or at your sides. Hands can be palms up or palms down, whatever feels right for you.

Or you may choose to sit on a mat or carpet on the floor, perhaps resting your back against a wall. On the floor, you might find it comfortable to sit on a cushion or folded blanket with legs crossed, positioning your knees lower than your hips. Extending your legs out in front of you is fine as well. Your comfort is key. Feel free to move around to find the right position for you.

Lying-down meditation: When meditating in this position, the goal is typically to avoid falling sleep, so be thoughtful of where you lie down. If you have concerns that practicing on your bed or couch will lead to falling asleep, try stretching out on a yoga mat (or try a seated position instead). You may use a rolled-up blanket or small pillow to support your head or neck. While lying on your back, position your legs about hip width apart, and allow the feet to naturally fall open. Palms will face upward with arms comfortably at your sides. Another option to help support your lower back is to bend your knees with feet on the ground, or, with legs straight, place a rolled blanket or pillow under your knees.

Standing meditation: This is a nice option for people who spend a lot of the day sitting. It can be done by simply pushing yourself away from your desk and standing up, or walking to a quiet place nearby. If your physician has mentioned that moving more throughout the day could assist with your gut motility, standing meditation is an ideal tool. Standing and walking can also help speed up digestion; therefore, these types of meditation can feel great after eating a meal, prior to returning to your desk at work or school, or before lying down for the night.

Let's Practice Meditation

Begin for two minutes a day, and work up to ten minutes After a while, you may find yourself practicing for twenty to thirty minutes. You can read through this passage a few times to get the hang of it, then begin on your own. You can also record yourself reading it aloud, or ask a loved one to read it to you.

Seated or lying meditation: Begin seated on a chair or cushion in an upright, relaxed position, or comfortably lying down. Close your eyes, and begin to focus your attention on your breath. As you sit, feel the sensations of your body. Then move to awareness of any thoughts and feelings you may have. Allow the thoughts and feelings to come and go. Return your attention to your breath and your body. You may envision the thoughts, feelings, and sensations in your body as waves that are coming onto shore and then washing away. Be aware of the waves, and allow yourself to find stillness. Feel your breath. Let your attention focus on the sensation of the cool air coming into your nostrils as you inhale and the warm air moving out your mouth as you exhale. Notice the sensations in the nose or your throat as you inhale. As you exhale, feel your chest or stomach gently fall. Relax into this pattern of breathing, and notice how the rest of your body begins to respond. Invite a stillness into your abdomen. Picture it calming and soothing the digestive tract. Let your breath fall into a natural rhythm, and concentrate on how it feels in your body. Continue to let any sensations, thoughts, or feelings come and go like waves in the background, as if you were at a beach. If your attention gets carried away from your breathing by one of the waves, simply notice this, and then redirect your attention to your breath. Whatever wave carried your attention away, perhaps name it softly— "worry," "cramping," "the future"—and then let it go. Sometimes you will be able to quickly return your focus to your breathing; at other times you will require more time. This is completely normal.

Standing meditation: With feet shoulder width apart, close your eyes if it feels comfortable to do so. Allow your body to release stress simply by imagining the tension evaporating into the space around you. Let your knees bend slightly. Place your hands on your stomach with one hand on top of the other. Notice the warmth of your hands and how that warmth is carried onto your belly. Feel your inhalations and exhalations and how they move through your body. Imagine your digestive system being soothed with your breath. Allow your body to be rooted into the ground with your exhalations. Notice what it's like to feel the full support of the ground under you. Envision your energy moving through your body, lifting out through the crown of your head with each inhalation. Notice a comfortable warmth moving through your digestive tract with each exhalation, calming and soothing your entire digestive system with each breath you take.

4. Grounding Yourself in Nature

If you close your eyes and envision yourself in a calm place, you might find your mind drifting to someplace in nature. Our body and mind can benefit immensely from being outside. As humans, we have evolved from spending most of our day outside to spending most of it inside. In light of this massive shift, being one with nature doesn't come easily to most people. We have to work at it, and when we do, we can reap tremendous health benefits. A growing body of literature points to the benefits of earthing, also known as grounding, in which a person connects bodily with the earth to stabilize themselves through the earth's natural electric charges. The beach is a perfect place to try grounding. Take off your shoes and feel the sand beneath your feet. Other research points to the benefits of forest bathing, spending time in the fresh air of a forest environment as opposed to an urban environment, where pollution often affects air quality. Regardless of how you want to spend your time outdoors, begin with a commitment to get fresh air daily. Work your way toward thirty minutes each day.

Let's Practice Grounding

Take a walk: Dress for the weather. If it is hot, take your shoes off and feel the benefits of your toes touching the earth. If you have limited mobility in your legs or are in a wheelchair, reach for something natural, such as a flower or leaf, and connect with it, using all the senses available to you. If it is cold, bundle up and get moving. Your body will know what it is able to do. (Accumulate the necessary cold-weather apparel. Having boots, rain gear, and gloves on hand removes the barrier of getting yourself out the door.) And if it is one of those perfect days—neither too hot nor too cold—embrace it!

Move and meditate: The beauty of meditation is that it can be done wherever and whenever you want to bring attention to the present moment. In a walking meditation, you keep your eyes open and bring awareness to your surroundings. This is particularly helpful if you are being bothered by unhelpful or anxious thoughts. Shift your focus from the swirling thoughts to what is happening during your walk. A lovely, proactive stress management strategy is to plan for a walking meditation in a place that genuinely brings you comfort and peace, be it a park, beach, country road, or hiking path. Let the beauty of that place guide your meditation. Wherever you are, you will begin to shift your attention to your pace and how you are holding your body, without feeling pressured to make any changes. Keep walking and observing the style of your walk. Then focus your attention on the setting around you.

Explore different routes: Escaping to a nature preserve is probably not possible every day. Just go where you can, and change it up! This may mean walking your child to school or to the bus stop in the morning, strolling in a parking lot midday, or walking around the block in the evening. Make a date with a caring friend or family member, and look for places to explore on a weekend or evening. As you seek out new places for walks or hikes, you create new habits that can connect you to others as well.

5. Accepting Strong Emotions

When an emotional storm hits, anchoring in the present moment will help you cope with difficult situations. When we experience stress, as we all know very well, our body jumps into the GI stress cycle. Stress overload can happen when we are inundated by a heavy situation. You can feel your body responding with an increased heart rate, short and shallow breathing, stomach cramping, and abdominal pain and bloating. Acknowledge the strong emotions you are having. The goal of this practice isn't necessarily to make the stress go away but to root yourself in the present moment to help you handle it. That way, you avoid getting swept away by racing thoughts or feelings. In his e-book *The Single Most Powerful Technique for Extreme Fusion*, Dr. Russ Harris, an expert in acceptance and commitment therapy (ACT), points out that dropping an anchor doesn't make a storm go away—it just holds the boat steady. What a powerful metaphor! The storm comes and goes in its own time, but you can learn techniques that will make you less likely to be overwhelmed by it.

Let's Practice Accepting Strong Emotions

Begin by silently and kindly acknowledging to yourself what emotions you are feeling. Perhaps you feel hurt, fearful, irritable, anxious. Begin to accept these emotions. Give yourself a few moments to do this.

You can then start to anchor yourself by pushing your feet into the ground. Feel your feet pressing hard into the floor. Straighten your back. If sitting in a chair, sit up straight. If you are in a hallway, you can stand up straight against a wall. Anchor your body against the chair or wall. Notice what this feels like. Press your fingertips together, or stretch your arms out wide. Shrug your shoulders.

Continue to acknowledge the painful, challenging, or difficult thoughts and feelings that are present with you in this moment. Accept that these thoughts and feelings are happening. Also recognize that there is a body around the thoughts and feelings, a body that you have some control over. A body that you can move. Come back to noticing what your body is doing. Notice your hands, your feet, your back. Continue to press your feet down and ground yourself.

Now look around you. Locate five things that you can see. Then focus on three or four things you can hear. Next, notice what you are doing in this moment. You can observe that you are calming yourself in a time of stress. Then come back to the present moment by returning your awareness to where you are and how your body feels.

Hopefully you now have greater focus and self-regulation. You can ask yourself, "What is important for me to focus on next?" We are better able to concentrate when we feel less overwhelmed by our stress.

As you begin to incorporate these skills into your daily life, you will start to master the goal of having fewer physical responses to the happenings around you. Paying attention to your body's signs when under stress creates opportunities for activating your parasympathetic system—yay, relaxation response! You have the power to decrease tension when the alarms are going off. Perhaps you can already reflect on a time when you found diaphragmatic breathing helpful in calming a tense stomach. Self-awareness can provide a measure of control when it feels like the train is running off the tracks and IBS symptoms are worsening. Simply knowing that you have skills to slow the train can alleviate stress. Now that you have better awareness of your emotional signs, we can move on to the cognitive ones: how to stop and shift negative, counterproductive thoughts.

CHAPTER 3

CHANGE YOUR THOUGHTS, CHANGE YOUR GUT

1. *No one else seems to be running to the bathroom five times before this exam. It's not fair!*
2. *If I didn't have IBS, I'd be way more productive.*
3. *Everyone else seems to have so much more energy than me. What is my problem?*
4. *My kids see me struggling with my health. I'm sure that can't be good for them.*
5. *I dread eating. I know my day is shot as soon as I have my first couple of bites.*

Do any of these types of thoughts sound familiar? How we think has a tremendous impact on how we feel physically and emotionally. Our thoughts can help us feel confident and capable of handling the difficult situations stemming from IBS, or they can bully us into believing we are incapable of a challenge, and therefore it's best to avoid one. As you continue down this road of empowering yourself to manage digestive distress, you are also learning why IBS can be so complicated. It usually isn't just one thing that can instigate how your bowels behave. Think back to what happened at the onset of your last stomach rumble and grumble. Not only can symptoms generate a GI stress cycle; often the feelings that are part of the cycle trigger unhelpful, automatic thoughts. "Here we go again. This is so frustrating and is going to ruin my morning!" The thoughts, or cognitions, may enter so quickly that we don't stop to question whether they are actually true.

Your thoughts play a part in your health whether you are closely aware of them or not. It's time to dive into the incredible power of the mind and the automatic thoughts that arise in all kinds of situations we encounter throughout the day. This chapter will teach you ways to shift the negative thought patterns that pop up when IBS strikes and to move into more helpful ways of thinking.

BRAIN BITE: COUNTERACT BULLYING THOUGHTS

- *Instead of:* No one else seems to be running to the bathroom five times before this exam. It is not fair!
  Try: Exams are stressful for most. I know that the power of test prep for me includes studying and self-care.

- *Instead of:* If I didn't have IBS, I'd be way more productive.
  Try: IBS is a bummer, but I can manage it! I am capable and resilient.

- *Instead of:* Everyone else seems to have so much more energy than me. What is my problem?
  Try: My energy level hasn't been quite where I want it. I'm going to be more mindful of my nutrition, sleep, and stress.

- *Instead of:* My kids see me struggling with my health. I'm sure that can't be good for them.
  Try: When I'm not feeling well, it's important to communicate to the kids that it is okay to take time for healing. No one is any good to others if they aren't taking care of themselves.

- *Instead of:* I dread eating. I know my day is shot as soon as I have my first couple of bites.
  Try: I'm going to try foods that are gentle on my stomach when I need to, and focus on one meal at a time. I can't predict the future.

CBT FOR IBS

Principles of cognitive behavioral therapy (CBT) are immensely helpful in the management of IBS. The research on psychological therapies is advancing, even taking us closer to identifying biomarkers for IBS. A recent joint study from researchers at the University of California, Los Angeles, and the University of Buffalo produced extremely promising results, demonstrating that a specific type of CBT focused on teaching individuals processing skills was able to modify key components of the brain-gut-microbiome axis in some people with IBS. Interestingly, study participants reported improvements in their GI symptoms, which corresponded with actual biological changes in their microbiome and brain function. This knowledge advances us toward identifying a precise gut microbiome "signature" that characterizes who will respond most favorably to CBT. Talk about progress!

The GI cognitive behavioral therapy model shown in Figure 4 demonstrates that how you *think* affects how you feel *emotionally*, which affects how you *behave*, which affects how you *feel physically*. It is important to note that changing any of these factors can influence the others. For example, you could change your thoughts pertaining to a physical sensation ("This stomachache is uncomfortable, but I can manage it and proceed with my day"), or you could change your behavior (get up off the couch, go for a short walk outside, and assess how that affects your discomfort). Each can have a positive impact on the sensations in your body. Understanding the interrelated nature of your thoughts, feelings, and behaviors can help you make meaningful changes for your IBS.

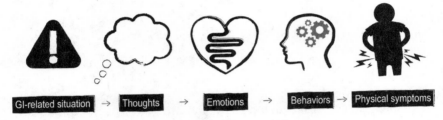

Figure 4: The GI Cognitive Behavioral Therapy Model

CHECK IN WITH YOUR COGNITIVE SIGNS

As clinicians working in the field of gastroenterology, we hear common frustrations from our patients. You, too, may find there are some things you tell yourself over and over during a flare-up. "IBS is ruining my life." "I'm never going to make it on time; what is the point of even going?" "How will I ever pass this class if I spend hours in the bathroom?" "I can't burden my friends with my dietary restrictions again, so I will just bail." It takes practice to slow down and observe when you are traveling along these familiar—and perhaps self-fulfilling—negative self-talk pathways. Like noticing when your body is telling you to take a drink of water and catch your breath during exercise, catching these exhausting thoughts can serve as a warning sign that it would be best to pause, take a few deep breaths, and come up with a new way of thinking.

CBT skills offer you ways to:

1. *Catch* your unhelpful automatic thoughts.
2. *Check* them for accuracy, or assess whether they are help- ing or hurting your current situation or stressor.
3. *Change* the thoughts to more advantageous ways of think- ing and behaving.

In CBT, we call these the three Cs. We like to tell patients to give themselves a pep talk by chanting, "Catch it, check it, change it!" It can also be helpful to systematically monitor your thoughts by writing them down in a thought record (a blank one is included in the Resources section). Using the Mind Your Gut Thought Record, you can observe your feelings, track your current thoughts regard- ing a particular stressor, and challenge those thoughts to find a more balanced way of managing your situation. Psychology experts call this cognitive restructuring, and it is a critical skill for improving the management of your IBS.

Cognitive restructuring typically leads to a decrease in GI dis- tress by mitigating the automatic thoughts that can flood us in the face of stress. Unless we become aware of this happening, the seem- ingly instantaneous thoughts often go unchecked for accuracy and can lead to a deluge of anxiety or distress. Let's see how quickly it happens.

Emma is invited to the movies with a friend. As her friend gives her the details for their outing, Emma begins to think:

- I'm probably going to have to run to the bathroom all the time.
- I will be a huge distraction to the other people in the theater if I must get up and use the loo.

- I'm sure my friend will be embarrassed if she has to wait a long time for me to return.
- I'll miss half the movie and won't know what's going on.
- Going to the movies is the absolute worst idea, and I really shouldn't agree to it.

All these habitual and unconscious thoughts occur in a matter of seconds. Unless they get checked for accuracy, what is the likely outcome of this situation? Either Emma will back out, or she will go and spend the entire time worrying. Avoidance and anxiety will rule again in the face of unpredictability. The goal of IBS therapies is to manage symptoms and allow for a more complete life. This is where CBT can help.

Certain common types of thinking traps or cognitive distortions occur when people feel stressed. Emma experienced several in the minutes she was on the phone with her friend. These included catastrophizing, mental filtering, fortune-telling, and all-or-nothing thinking. If you see yourself in one or more of these patterns, don't blame yourself. We all periodically fall victim to our internal naysayer. No one can think rationally 100 percent of the time. CBT is about learning how to recognize cognitive distortions and overcome them by shifting to another, more constructive mindset.

CATCH AND CHANGE YOUR COGNITIVE DISTORTIONS

Distorted thoughts:

- Tend to be beliefs or habitual patterns of thinking that we have about the world.
- Tend to be false, inaccurate, and exaggerated.
- Are often accompanied by uncomfortable emotions.

- Can have an impact on our bodily sensations, causing butterflies in the stomach, tension, short breathing, flashes of heat or sweating, and increased heart rate.
- May increase symptoms of anxiety and depression as well as GI distress.

Start paying attention to your thoughts, and see if you can catch yourself engaging in any of the following common distortions:

Catastrophic thinking: You believe that a situation is worse than it really is and feel helpless.

Example: "I am completely disabled by this diarrhea, and if I leave the house and can't find a bathroom, I will surely have an accident. IBS ruins my whole life."

Change the thoughts: "I'm having diarrhea right now, but I can help calm it down. Let me practice some diaphragmatic breathing and see how I feel in an hour."

All-or-nothing thinking: You view things in absolutes, extremes, and black-or-white terms. There is no gray area.

Example: "I don't feel great. I'm canceling all plans and not leaving the house for the day."

Change the thoughts: "There have been times when I didn't feel great, and I was still able to make it through my day. I think I'll take it one task at a time and see how I feel. I'll start with dropping the kids off at school."

Mental filtering: You focus on a single negative detail and dwell on it to the point that it colors the entire situation in an unpleasant light.

Example: You gave a presentation at work, and your boss said you nailed it. However, your stomach gurgled throughout, and you thought the team heard it. "All I can think about now that the presentation is done is how everyone must have heard that gurgling. How unprofessional. What if they thought I was passing gas? Can this day just be over?"

Change the thoughts: Work to shift your focus to the positive aspects of your presentation. Remind yourself that your boss gave positive feedback. Ask yourself how others would respond to your interpretation of the situation. If you feel they would challenge it, explore what you think they may say to you. "Even if my symptoms were acting up, I was well prepared, got great feedback, and I'm going to let myself sit in the success of that presentation."

Shoulds, oughts, musts: You experience frustration or guilt when you don't achieve what you've told yourself you should.

Example: "I should have known better than to eat that. Now my stomach is a wreck. I must not have done a good job listening to my dietitian. I ought to just cancel the next appointment."

Change the thoughts: "I am 'shoulding' on myself right now. My dietitian told me that I don't have to be perfect with these nutritional strategies. This is a bit of a setback, but I'll get back to following her suggestions this evening. I will be okay!"

Fortune-telling: You negatively predict the future without actually considering facts or the odds of that outcome.

Example: "Nothing I try for managing these symptoms will work. It is time to leave the house, and here comes pain, gas, and bloating. It never fails—I have the urge to go and nothing comes out. I'm sure as soon as I'm out the door, that's when it will hit. Especially if I am nowhere near a bathroom."

Change the thoughts: Consider possibility versus probability. Although it is possible that your negative prediction may happen, what is the actual probability that it will? For example, if you fear that you could have a bowel accident, calculate how many times in the last year you have had an accident. If you have never had an accident, then take note of the fact that 100 percent of the time in the last year you never had a bowel accident! If you have had one accident in the preceding 365 days, then 99.7 percent of the time in the last year, you did not have an accident. Instead of focusing on the amount of time a worry was successfully averted, we often dwell on the very unlikely possibility that it could happen. Another way to think about this is to consider the odds. If the probability that you would win the lottery were 99.7 percent, you'd buy a ticket, right? You would be feeling good about your chances and focused on how you will spend your winnings, not fixated on the 0.3 percent chance that you might not win. In the lottery of IBS, focus on the fact that more times than not you make it through the day without a bowel accident. The skills that you are learning now can give you a lot more confidence!

CBT THOUGHT RECORD: LET'S WORK THIS OUT ON PAPER

Keeping a thought record involves writing down and organizing your thoughts about a stressful situation so that you can more clearly identify and correct cognitive distortions. It's a helpful exercise when learning to implement CBT. As close to the onset of the stressor as you can, use the following questions and prompts to complete a thought record.

Where are you? Who are you with? Describe your surroundings when you had the thought.

What are your emotions or feelings? Describe one to three emotions or feelings you have about this stressor. Rate the intensity of each from 0 (not intense) to 100 (most intense).

Can you identify a negative automatic thought? What thought or thoughts were going through your mind at the time of the stressor? What memories came to mind?

What evidence supports that thought? What facts support the truthfulness or accuracy of the thought?

What evidence does not *support the thought?* Ask yourself worry-control questions (more about these later in the chapter) to aid in checking your thoughts. Am I jumping to negative conclusions? What experiences indicate that this thought is not completely true? What would I tell a friend in this situation if they had the same thoughts?

What alternative thought or helpful perspective can you consider? Write a new thought that takes into consideration the evidence for and against your automatic thought. You've caught and checked your thoughts; now it is time to change them to something more accurate and helpful.

What are your emotions or feelings in this new moment? How do you feel about the situation now? Reconsider the intensity, from 0 to 100. Some feelings may be completely gone or significantly reduced in severity, and new feelings may have replaced them (e.g., confident, calm, relieved).

Let's go back to Emma, who was contemplating whether to go to the movies or not. How could a thought record assist her? Figure 5 shows an example of a thought record that she might complete as soon as she hangs up with her friend.

Completing a thought record at the onset of your discomfort can help prevent you from getting swept away by the GI stress cycle. It also puts you in the mindset of addressing your stress with confidence rather than avoiding the situation. See the Resources section for a blank copy of the Mind Your Gut Thought Record for your own use. Use the prompts to guide your process.

FACING THE URGE TO AVOID ACTIVITIES

If Emma hadn't taken some time to change her initial automatic thoughts regarding the invitation to the movies, she likely would have stayed home. The drive to avoid is fueled by anxiety. Though it's tempting to skip activities for fear of an IBS flare-up, guess what? Avoidance is our enemy in many cases. Did you know that the act of avoiding gives a false sense of control, which actually increases symptoms of anxiety and can worsen how you feel about yourself? Understanding how this all works is helpful. As you become able to

MIND YOUR GUT **THOUGHT RECORD**

Where are you? Who are you with?
At home on the phone with my friend, then alone after the call.

What are your emotions or feelings?
Rate the intensity from 0–100.
Anxious (75)
Frustrated (60)

Negative automatic thoughts:
Going to the movies is a very bad idea.
I'll be embarrassed by the number of times I need to get up and go to the bathroom.
My friend will be annoyed with me.

Evidence that supports your thoughts:
There was that time a year ago when I was in the bathroom for almost an entire movie. It was terribly embarrassing.

Evidence that does not support your thoughts:
I've been to the movies a few times without any IBS symptoms and enjoyed myself.
This is a good friend, and she would likely be understanding regardless of my needs.

Alternative thought or helpful perspective:
I am going to use my skills before going to the movies and plan that I will be okay!
If I get myself all worked up before anything happens that won't help. I am excited to spend time with my friend.

Emotions or feelings in this moment.
Reconsider intensity from 0–100.
Anxious (25)
Excited (70)
Confident (65)

Figure 5. Emma's Thought Record for a Stressful Situation

recognize some of the habitual thought patterns that tend to happen in times of IBS distress, you can use these opportunities to pivot in a way that lessens anxiety. Let's look at another example.

Mira wakes up on the morning of her first presentation at work. She has prepared for this presentation for several weeks and had been feeling confident about it earlier in the week. However, she's feeling some stomach cramps and has run to the bathroom twice while trying to get her day going. The way she thinks through managing her morning may significantly affect how the rest of the day goes.

Path number one: "This is really bad. I've had it happen before where my stomach keeps me in the bathroom, and I just know my colleagues are thinking there is something wrong with me. It is so embarrassing. I'm sure this doesn't happen to my boss. My IBS ruins everything. I can't possibly deal with the criticism and the chance that I'll have diarrhea at work. I'm going to call in sick today and postpone this presentation."

Path number two: "Ugh. This is frustrating, and I know the stress of this presentation is probably kicking up some nerves in my body. Even though my stomach has caused problems by making me have to spend extra time in the bathroom before, I have been working on some strategies to calm things down, and I've got this! It is normal for people to get butterflies before a presentation. I'm prepared. I got great feedback from my colleagues as I put it together, and I am not going to let my anxiety and stomach stop me. Even if I feel a bit off this morning, I am sure I will feel better once the presentation gets started."

There is no question that walking down path two can take guts and practice. Becoming aware of our thoughts and their impact on our decision-making—and then changing them—requires work! Path one is easier. But calling in sick and postponing the presentation will not actually help Mira at all.

If Mira takes path one, IBS wins again. Those uncomfortable stomach sensations will have triggered fear and undercut her confidence that she could handle her physical health. People with IBS tend to have increased hypervigilance (the brain pays extra attention to every sensation in the digestive system) and hypersensitivity (the brain has a difficult time calming the signals from the gut, and therefore senses more in the intestines than it should be picking up on). This leads to heightened autonomic arousal during periods of stress (heart rate increases, breathing becomes short and shallow, muscles tense up, stomach distress worsens . . .). Definitely uncomfortable! Another player driving path one is a type of anxiety that people with IBS experience: visceral anxiety or GI symptom–specific anxiety, which you learned about in the last chapter. With it, the response to a GI sensation can be out of proportion to the actual severity of the symptoms, contributing to increased pain. Then additional scenarios can happen.

Path one, scenario A: Mira remains home, and the symptoms persist. She continues thinking about how bad it would have been if she were at work and feeling this way. She is also extremely angry with herself that she can't give the presentation and worries about whether this could hurt her career. While running back and forth to the bathroom, she anticipates her colleagues thinking she is unreliable and assumes that she won't be asked to present anytime soon.

Path one, scenario B: She is home and feels better almost immediately. Now the stress of potentially having her IBS symptoms worsen at work is over. She perceives that her body is "safely" near a restroom if needed, and therefore it calms down. However, this is a false sense of security. The anxiety will likely come back and be problematic in the future. Anxiety and worry are rooted in situations that are uncontrollable or unpredictable. The most effective way to manage anxiety is to face it head-on. Teach your body and mind that you can manage even the most uncomfortable situations, whether related to your IBS or to other areas of life. Let's look a bit closer at the pitfalls of avoidance.

STOP OVERAVOIDANCE

For decades, we have worked with people to help them face their anxiety and get back to the enjoyable things they have allowed IBS to prevent them from doing. The spontaneity of allowing someone else to plan an outing; eating at restaurants; driving long distances; traveling in trains, planes, or boats; sitting in certain locations while in public (a concert, the theater, your child's recital)—you could probably name a dozen more activities your gut has steered you away from.

If missing out on life feels familiar, you are not alone. Many people with IBS often have a lot of worry or anxiety about their GI symptoms and how they may play out in public. Research has shown that anxiety has a bigger impact on your health-related quality of life than the actual GI symptom severity.

In reality, avoiding situations for fear of how your gut may behave is counterproductive. Why? Because your *thoughts* create that fear. Often those thoughts are catastrophic, based on strong beliefs that something unfortunate will happen and negative predictions about the outcome. You allow your mind to limit your ability to embrace life's adventures or daily opportunities before you even leave the house.

Catastrophic thinking is a (misguided) attempt to control the possibility of something uncomfortable happening. Dr. Riehl likes to point out how unfair this is to your brain. The anxiety makes the brain work to come up with all kinds of "solutions" to problems that haven't actually happened yet. This isn't to say that all anxiety is bad. Some anxiety can help you adequately prepare, such as noticing where a bathroom is when you arrive at a new location, keeping some Imodium easily accessible when traveling, or choosing a gentle meal if you've recently had a flare of symptoms. There is merit in the military slogan "proper preparation prevents poor performance" (the five Ps). However, overthinking a problem and solution will likely put your brain in overdrive.

If you are anxious, the mind may take you to past experiences that didn't go as you would have liked, reminding you that, yes indeed, something embarrassing could happen again. At the same time, the mind is also vaulting into the future trying to find a solution that will be difficult to execute, because the event hasn't, in fact, occurred. All this ramps up physical sensations—hello, fight-or-flight response. If you aren't aware of the benefits of riding things out and trusting that you are capable of coping with unknowns, you will do everything you can to make the uncomfortable thoughts and feelings go away. In comes the temporary advantage of avoidance: "If I just don't do it/go there/eat that, I won't have to deal with the potential GI mess." But in the long run, it actually worsens the load of life with IBS.

BRAIN BITE: REAL CHANGE TAKES TIME

Realizing that it is time to make some adjustments in your thought processes can feel overwhelming. Maybe you have been thinking in certain anxious ways for as long as you can remember. Change is not expected to happen overnight. It will take practice and making small adjustments to the way you approach difficult situations. Over time, this can have a big impact on your confidence in managing life with IBS. Don't worry, we will provide you with the tools to begin making these mindset shifts.

When our intestines seem uncontrollable, we naturally seek things to control. This typically includes one's diet. In an effort to prevent inconvenient or embarrassing symptoms, some IBS patients over-restrict their foods. Unfortunately, unnecessary restriction has been shown to lower quality of life and make living with IBS harder. As you read through the nutrition chapters, Kate will enlighten you on how to adjust your diet for good symptom control without the need for major limitations or constraints.

DIGESTIBLE DETAIL: BE FOOD-CURIOUS

Following an elimination diet can be quite helpful to keep IBS symptoms in check. But a very restrictive diet has been shown to increase risk of social isolation and to lower quality of life. When choosing a change in diet as a way to reduce digestive distress in IBS, remain curious about foods, and, with guidance from your health-care team, periodically reintroduce different foods to test your tolerance. Important reminder: Your tolerance to foods can change over time!

ARE YOU MISSING OUT ON ANYTHING?

If you feel you are missing out on aspects of life you once enjoyed because of fears related to your IBS, let's change that. Unfortunately, it's possible that you have been avoiding life's pleasures for so long that you don't even realize what you are missing. Let's start down the road to change by first taking an assessment of common negative thoughts that drive avoidance.

Going for a walk or run: "I've had a few accidents on runs before. It is the most mortifying situation in life."

Change the thoughts: "Today, I'll go as far as my body will allow."

Air travel: "What if I must go to the bathroom while the seat belt sign is on?! I would surely have an accident."

Change the thoughts: "I will give myself time to use the bathroom before getting on the plane, then once seated, I'll practice diaphragmatic breathing to distract myself and calm my mind and stomach."

Eating at a loved one's house: "My stomach is so sensitive that it is embarrassing to list all the things I can't eat. It's too much of a burden."

Change the thoughts: "It is okay to let those who care about me know about my dietary preferences. I would want someone to feel comfortable at my house. I'm sure they feel the same way about me."

Happy hour with friends or colleagues: "I never know what my stomach will be like by the end of a workday, and I don't want to cancel all the time."

Change the thoughts: "I can't predict how I will feel in the future. It is nice to have something to look forward to at the end of a long day, and I can make adjustments to the plans if needed."

Staying at a friend's house or sharing a hotel room: "There is only one bathroom, and there is no way I could let them know what goes on in there!"

Change the thoughts: "If I am close enough with someone to be invited to share a space, surely they will be compassionate about my bathroom habits."

Carpooling: "I could never let someone else drive because I often need to stop to use the bathroom and I wouldn't want to hold them up. It's also embarrassing to say I need to stop when no one else does, especially multiple times."

Change the thoughts: "Instead of avoiding this entirely, I can allow myself to take it one car trip at a time."

Going to a concert or show: "The line for the bathroom is always a mile long, and I cannot get in a stall fast enough."

Change the thoughts: "Strangers can be kind. If I really needed to go, I can ask to move to the front of the line. I know the key is to keep myself calm."

Dating, sex: "There is no way I could let a significant other hear, smell, or see what happens when my symptoms are bad. They would be repulsed. I would be humiliated."

Change the thoughts: "As I get to know someone, I will remind myself that I am more than IBS. The right person for me will embrace that and accept all of me."

Working: "Prior to the pandemic, I hated everything about going to work. The commute, the lack of privacy in the bathroom, embarrassment if I passed gas. Now there is no way I can go back to the office, and my boss is not happy with me."

Change the thoughts: "Having flexibility to work from home is important to me, and maybe there are opportunities for hybrid work. Either way, now I've got tools to navigate things that I used to avoid. I can put my coping skills to use when I head to work."

Medical procedures: "My doctor wants me to get a colonoscopy, and I am paralyzed with fear to go under anesthesia. So I just don't schedule it."

Change the thoughts: "I can do hard things. I'm going to focus on the suggestions in the Colonoscopy-Coping Prep Kit and get that procedure done! I will feel relief knowing I have managed an aspect of my health that is controllable." (Find the prep kit in Appendix II if you have been postponing a colonoscopy.)

These types of thoughts, especially the ones regarding some of life's most pleasurable activities, lead to false beliefs that if you avoid activities, things will be okay. But by doing so, you are not allowing yourself to live your life to the fullest. And everyone deserves that.

TECHNIQUES TO GET YOU TO YES

The next several strategies are going to help you say yes instead. Some of the suggestions for overcoming avoidance are from the newest science related to the use of CBT for IBS and involve a process called interoceptive exposure. The techniques focus on reducing anxiety and avoidance by repeated exposure to visceral sensations (actual sensations in the gut, such as stomach clenching or fullness). In a therapy setting, a psychologist will work with the person to face feared sensations and situations using strategies such as delaying defecation, tightening the stomach to produce gut sensations, or eating foods that have been restricted or anxiety-provoking. The interoceptive exposure interventions are aimed at alleviating GI-specific anxiety by deliberately inducing the sensations that drive worry. Interoceptive exposure weakens the fear response, allowing you to shift your attention to your coping skills. You can reap some of the benefits of this technique by directly facing your IBS fears. Here's how to create a mindset for success.

Coping Statements

How you think affects how you feel. Optimistic thoughts have the power to calm you when you begin to feel those uncomfortable GI sensations that drive panic. Instead of avoiding the discomfort, you can repeat a single statement or give yourself time to come up with the mindset shift that settles you. At the same time, you may find it helpful to check in on your breathing (and relax your muscles too).

Coping statements offer you a starting place for calm. First, practice saying the following words to yourself while in a relaxed, balanced state of mind, which will enable you to internalize the messages. As you begin to believe the statements, you will eventually find that even in seemingly out-of-control situations, you *are* in control of something: your thoughts. You will grow confident in your capability to handle whatever situation is before you. Take a snapshot of this list with your phone to refer to as needed. Eventually you may find yourself automatically repeating some of the statements when you need them most.

- I can handle uncomfortable things.
- This is not an emergency. I can come up with a plan.
- I choose to be calm.
- I can do hard things.
- No one has died from embarrassment. I will persevere no matter what.
- I am not in danger. These feelings in my body will pass.
- I can handle this.
- This is not the worst thing that can happen to me.
- This is anxiety, and I am not going to let it get worse.
- Nothing terrible is going to happen to me right now.
- I am safe.
- These thoughts are not helpful. I can think differently.
- Even though I don't feel great, anxiety will not hurt me.
- I acknowledge that this doesn't feel good, but it won't last forever.
- I am capable of managing this discomfort.
- This is my opportunity to use my coping skills to manage this situation.
- I deserve to feel better.
- I've survived things like this in the past, and I can do it again.
- I can take as much time as I need to let this pass. It will pass.
- The feelings in my body are not comfortable, but I can accept this.
- Even while anxious, I can deal with this situation.

People often find that gaining the ability to observe their thoughts and make adjustments is empowering. How about this for a visual: Imagine teaching a rambunctious dog (whom you love greatly) how to walk on a leash. At first, the dog may be running all over the place. If you do not assert your dominance over the dog, it will never learn. You must keep a tight grip on the leash and pull the pup in. You give the dog a stiff look, a firm grip, and an assertive command to "Sit." It feels good to take control and lead that dog down the road. If you don't maintain your position of power, the dog will pull you all over the street.

Envision pulling in that metaphorical leash when your rambunctious and unhelpful thoughts are jumping around. You are the master of your thinking—let's reel it in!

Stopping Thoughts

As we know, an avalanche of negative thoughts can be overwhelming. Sometimes we need to just end the thoughts in order to employ some of our other CBT skills. The STOP technique can be used to halt your unhelpful thoughts and defuse a stressful situation. It's a mindfulness-based skill to help you gain perspective in the moment and determine next steps in your coping. Think, "STOP."

Stop: Disrupt your thoughts by saying, in your mind or out loud, "*Stop*." Pause what you are doing.

Take a breath: Focus your attention on your breathing for six breaths. Shift to diaphragmatic breathing (page 57) if you notice GI distress.

Observe: Notice your thoughts, feelings, and physical sensations. Tune into these sensations, and let whatever is occurring happen for the moment.

Proceed: In the present moment, decide what you and your body need. What is one thing you can control and focus on? Choose one small step, and move forward to act on it.

Worry-Control Questions

Worry-control questions can be used alone or while filling out a thought record. They help you check the accuracy of your thoughts while also demonstrating your ability to cope, even if the situation is really difficult. It can be helpful to keep these questions handy while you learn this skill. (Take another picture on your phone.) While not all the questions will be applicable in every situation, it is likely that some of them will be very valuable in terms of helping you shift your mindset. You can ask yourself:

- Am I overestimating the likelihood that something bad will happen?
- Am I catastrophizing right now?
- What is the worst-case scenario here? Could I deal with it?
- Who is someone that might be able to help me right now?
- Am I minimizing my ability to cope with an unexpected situation?
- Does worrying about this situation make it better?
- Can I cope with X minutes or days of stress or discomfort until this resolves?
- Have I been able to handle things like this in the past? What did I do?
- Do I know other people who have been in similar stressful situations?
- What is one small step I can take right now to feel better?
- What would I tell a friend in this situation?

Answering that last question can really be eye-opening. People with IBS tend to place pressure and guilt on themselves. If you have significant worry over inconveniencing a friend or loved one about needing to stop and use a bathroom, or to make dietary accommodations, try taking yourself out of the picture. When you pretend the roles are reversed, you realize that you would never be so hard on a friend in your situation. If a friend were talking to themselves the way you are talking to yourself, you would do everything in your power to put their mind at ease. If a friend were struggling, you would spend time to come up with a constructive and kind way to support them. We often fail to allow ourselves the same grace we give to others or to speak to ourselves with kindness. Being your own worst critic and holding yourself to a higher standard than you do your friends can be tremendously damaging. Speak to yourself with the same compassion that you have for others.

BRAIN BITE: BE YOUR OWN BEST FRIEND

Talk to yourself like you would a good friend. You are allowed to treat yourself with compassion, love, and respect.

Constructive Worry

Have you ever laid your head on the pillow knowing that you could really, really use a good night's sleep? Then your brain perks up and recognizes that the lights are off, it's nice and quiet, and therefore it's the perfect time to worry about everything! "What if I wake up with a stomachache? Gosh, I probably shouldn't have eaten that at dinner tonight. I have so much on my to-do list this week; I am never going to get it all done. Did I lock the door? I really need to get to sleep. I should have done a better job meal planning this week. The teacher said that my kid was coughing a lot in class today. I can't afford to take more time off for a sick day for them; I never know when I'll need it for my IBS. Ugh, my stomach is starting to hurt, I think I better try to go to the bathroom . . ."

In their book *Quiet Your Mind and Get to Sleep: Solutions to Insomnia for Those with Depression, Anxiety, or Chronic Pain,* Drs. Colleen Carney and Rachel Manber share a fantastic problem-solving strategy called constructive worry. The goal is to decrease the anxiety that can creep up at night and ruin your restful ZZZs. Much of the stress related to IBS is best addressed by slowing down and taking time to apply the proper coping strategy in the moment. If you are someone who has sleep disruptions due to anxiety and worry, this is the technique for you.

When do we do our best thinking? When we are well rested. When we have someone to talk with. When we can change the scenery or take time to do another task and come back to the issue. Generally speaking, the middle of the night is not a time that sets us up for success. At night, our body and our mind want to be sleeping. Struggling with sleep generates frustration, muscle tension, and increased stress hormones, all of which make sleep even more difficult. You are therefore unlikely to solve your problems in this scenario. Constructive worry allows you to manage problems in a much more effective environment, away from your bed. As you practice this skill, over time you will find that you have less to worry about when your head hits the pillow, because you have already spent time in a productive mindset brainstorming solutions and making plans. You took care of the problem long before the sun went down. Even if the worries do sneak up, you can more confidently remind yourself that now is not the time to think about them. This reassurance lends itself to a more restful mindset, and you can ease yourself to sleep. Let's practice.

1. Several hours before bed (aim for after dinner, or at least two hours before you plan to go to bed), set aside ten minutes to focus on this exercise. We believe that writing out the exercise by hand can feel cathartic, but feel free to type if that is your jam. On the left side of

a piece of paper, create a column labeled "Concerns." The right side of the paper will house a column for "Solutions."

2. Think about things that typically keep you up at night. In the "Concerns" column, write down one to three (no more than three) of the worries that come to mind.

3. Next, think about possible solutions for each worry. These do not have to be overly detailed, just enough to show yourself that you are capable of coping. You may find that you already have a solution to an issue. You may realize that the solution will likely come with time. You may conclude that you will benefit from talking it through with someone else. Whatever comes to mind as you brainstorm solutions, write them down in the "Solutions" column. Do this for each of your worries.

4. Place the paper somewhere away from your bedroom, and return to the rest of your evening. Tell yourself that you worked hard at solving your problems, and allow yourself to let go of them for now.

5. When your head hits the pillow, if you begin to worry, catch those thoughts. You can remind yourself that you have already addressed the concern in the most constructive way possible. You have some solutions that you plan to work on in daylight hours. No more effort is required right now. Give yourself permission to release the worry for the night, and shift into relaxing your body and mind.

Once you get into the habit of using this skill, as you build confidence in your problem-solving, you will notice that it actually helps lessen your daytime anxiety as well. You are then able to hit the hay feeling satisfied that your busy brain can recharge.

CONTROLLABLE VERSUS UNCONTROLLABLE STRESS: WHY IT MATTERS

Let's focus a little more on effective problem-solving, because it is such an important skill in stress management. Have you ever had a problem you were trying to solve, and it felt like you were stuck in mud, spinning your tires? Chances are you were applying a coping skill that didn't match the type of stressor you were trying to address. You were trying to fit a square peg in a round hole. No matter how you spin it, it's not going to work.

Identification of the kind of stress you are experiencing is a critical first step in problem-solving. If you dump all kinds of stress into one bucket and use the same coping skills all the time, you will find that you aren't always successful. There are certain types of coping skills for certain types of stress. For stressors that are controllable, we recommend use of problem-focused coping skills, and for stressors that are uncontrollable, we recommend emotion-focused coping skills. Based on the type of stressor, you will apply a certain type of coping skill.

In the same way that people with IBS use certain patterns of thinking, they tend to rely heavily on problem-focused coping regardless of the type of stress they are experiencing. We are often incredibly impressed by the skill of the people we work with when it comes to their ability to solve problems that have a potential resolution, no matter how complex that resolution may be. However, not all problems have a resolution—that is, not all problems are controllable stressors. That is where a completely different set of coping skills is needed. Enter emotion-focused coping for uncontrollable stressors. Let's look at some examples.

Controllable Stressors

- Scheduling a doctor's appointment
- Paying a bill
- Taking a test

- Completing a work assignment
- Choosing who you spend time with
- Taking prescribed medication

Uncontrollable Stressors

- The outcome of a medical procedure
- Travel delays or disruptions
- Availability of a bathroom
- Predicting when you will need a bathroom
- Waking up and not feeling well
- What other people think of you
- The weather

Problem-solving involves matching the right type of coping skill to the problem or stressor you are experiencing. To repeat, problem-focused coping is helpful for controllable stressors, while emotion-focused coping is helpful for managing stressors outside your control. As you will see, most people who have been living their lives trying to control their IBS are probably more comfortable using skills that seek an absolute resolution. That is what makes IBS so frustrating: it doesn't tend to allow for absolute resolution. However, when you learn that you have a much bigger bag of coping skills, the pressure to control becomes less intense, and you can enjoy the process of problem-solving—or at least feel more confident! Here are some examples of the two kinds of skills.

Problem-Focused Coping Skills

- Brainstorming to seek a resolution to the stressor
- Use of good time-management skills
- Practicing strong organizational skills (cue the to-do lists)
- Communicating directly with people so that you aren't making assumptions and can ensure that everyone is on the same

page (helpful with peers at school, colleagues at work, and family members at home)

Emotion-Focused Coping Skills

- Practicing meditation with regularity
- Daily relaxation
- Going for a walk or exercising
- Adopting an "it is what it is" attitude; practicing acceptance of an uncontrollable stressor
- Talking with a trusted companion or loved one
- Engaging in spiritual or faith-based practices
- Reminding yourself of your resilience (your ability to successfully adapt to difficult or challenging situations)

When you begin to realize that your ability to manage stress has a big impact on the outcome of an unfavorable situation, you feel more confident to handle whatever life tosses at you. Give yourself a silent (or out loud, whatever makes you happy) "Well done!" in recognition of your skills: "I can manage whatever comes my way!" If you don't feel a sense of accomplishment over how you are handling a situation, chances are you need to reevaluate the controllables and the uncontrollables and make sure you are applying the right type of coping strategy to the situation. Don't worry, this is a fluid process. Also, new or different stressors can unfold, and you will continue to apply the skills.

INTRUSIVE NEGATIVE THOUGHTS: IT IS OKAY TO NOT BE OKAY. HELP IS AVAILABLE!

Living with IBS can be difficult—especially if you feel hopeless about ever getting better. Even though we aim to provide you with a roadmap to better health, for some people, negative thoughts about themselves can be intrusive and downright scary. If you have thoughts of hurting yourself or of suicide, we want you to seek help immediately. Doing so is one of the most courageous steps you can take to feel better physically and emotionally. You are *not* alone, and now is the time to reach out for the support you deserve. Call a family member, friend, or doctor, and share how you feel and that you need help. Seek out a mental health professional, or ask a loved one to help you set up a first appointment. Here are some additional resources that are available right now:

- 988 Suicide & Crisis Lifeline: Dial 988 or 1-800-273-TALK (8255) (as of this publication).
- From your cell phone, text "HOME" to 741741 to connect with a crisis counselor.

If you find these cognitive behavioral strategies helpful and would like to take a deeper dive into this type of therapeutic work, check out the Resources for more information, including help locating a mental health professional. This book will not take the place of working with a clinician who specializes in CBT.

Your toolbox is growing. Are you beginning to feel the power of regulating your thoughts and feelings as you move through your day? You are seeing how your thoughts can be observed and changed to positively manage stressful situations. Slowing your thoughts can aid in slowing the body's panicky responses, which go hand in hand with GI distress. With a diverse set of psychological strategies at your disposal, you can expect continued improvements in your IBS symptoms. Now let's move on to our third anti-stress strategy.

CHAPTER 4

THE ROLE OF RELAXATION AND CARING FOR *YOU*

It's time to take stress reduction to the next level. As we've seen, your thoughts and emotions, if unchecked, can provoke or worsen uncomfortable sensations in the body—sending the GI stress cycle churning and keeping you in the bathroom. Just as you practiced paying attention to emotional signs of stress in Chapter 2 and cognitive signs in Chapter 3, you will now learn to tune in to the physical signs, or what we call sensation signs.

When we experience stress and anxiety, the body has a physiological response. The muscles can tense up, heart rate and blood pressure can escalate, and respiration can change (breathing speeds up or even slows down). People are often unaware of the signals that the body is delivering and thus completely miss opportunities to make a change before the body goes into overdrive. Recognizing those bodily sensations can help you de-escalate the tension that accompanies the stress of the day. Keep in mind that if you have tension in one part of your body (such as your shoulders, jaw, or hands), you are probably unnecessarily holding tension in your tummy too. Get ready for the art of deep relaxation.

CHECK IN WITH YOUR SENSATION SIGNS

At any given part of the day, you can notice things about your body. You can try it right now. Right this moment, pause and notice your shoulders. You may realize that you can pull them down away from your ears. This feels comfortable and provides a noticeable release of tension that you were unintentionally carrying. Now scan the rest of your body. Maybe you notice a cramp in your stomach. That's another sign. Pause and place your hand on your stomach. In your mind, acknowledge, "I felt that. I feel some tension in my stomach."

Continue scanning your body for tension. Maybe you can relax your jaw, neck, or hands. As your hand rests on your stomach, begin to release the tension from the other parts of your body, and notice how that feels.

As you take these moments to observe and acknowledge the signs from your body, you can choose to deepen your breath. Remember that you are able to calm your gut by calming other parts of your body. Take a moment of gratitude for your gut—for how it alerts you to check in with your body and make adjustments. As you remove your hands from your stomach, remind yourself to check in with yourself periodically. Release, relax, and return to your day with less tension and increased confidence.

CREATE THE RELAXATION HABIT

As you implement relaxation practices to get your IBS under control, aim to practice at the same time each day. This will assist you in creating healthy habits. Think about when would work best for you.

Remember to permit yourself grace and flexibility as you create your new routines.

- Set your morning alarm ten minutes early to begin the day with relaxation. As your gut settles, we hope you will continue to utilize the time for an ongoing daily practice.
- Schedule time for your self-care as if you were scheduling any other appointment. Plan the activity, and put it on your calendar.
- Set an alarm to practice one- to three-minute interventions (such as a mindful minute, sixty seconds of diaphragmatic breathing, a brief body scan) three times per day. We recommend picking times of the day when you consistently have downtime. For example, around mealtimes, while driving to work, and during your commute home.
- If you usually work from home, build in transition time in which to move your body in the midst of your usual schedule or between Zoom meetings. Make time for a brief relaxation practice, and give yourself a few moments to mindfully prepare for the next portion of your day.

Let's face it—being stressed doesn't just involve IBS. Living life in the best of circumstances still involves stressors; it's part of the human experience. But managing IBS-related stress can make a significant impact on your overall well-being. So make a commitment to give yourself time to practice relaxation. When you make it a habit, you can expect to see other health benefits, such as increased energy and productivity, reduced general anxiety, improved concentration and memory, increased self-confidence, reduced muscle tension, improved sleep, less daytime fatigue, and many more. There is lots to gain from consistently taking time to prioritize yourself.

HYPNOSIS FOR IBS (DON'T WORRY, THERE'S NO CLUCKING LIKE A CHICKEN)

Here's another popular and effective psychological intervention for IBS: hypnotherapy. (If you're skeptical, hear us out!) In fact, gut-directed hypnosis helps to restore the brain's everyday regulation of the GI tract and has one of the highest success rates of any treatment, based on many research studies. It can improve IBS symptoms and quality of life with results shown to last *years.*

Surprisingly, gut-directed hypnotherapy has been studied in the use of GI conditions, most commonly IBS, for nearly four decades. Numerous research trials have proved the benefits of using this technique with IBS patients no matter how symptoms present. That's right, regardless of diarrhea, constipation, or both, *over half of all people who have experienced inadequate relief with traditional medical treatment have had relief with hypnotherapy!* Further, gut-directed hypnotherapy has a better track record than the available medication options for the treatment of IBS (symptoms often return if you discontinue use of the medication). With hypnotherapy, 80 percent of those who experienced improvements in their symptoms at the end of treatment maintained those improvements for years after their last hypnosis session. Beyond bowel symptom relief, patients typically also experience many of the benefits provided by other relaxation and self-care strategies, including improvements in quality of life and decreases in non-GI symptoms such as headaches, backaches, urinary problems (e.g., frequent urination, urinary incontinence), and fatigue.

One of the biggest reasons why most people have not tried or even heard of gut-directed hypnotherapy for their IBS is due to limited access to trained GI mental health professionals who administer it. Fortunately, people can now access this treatment in reliable ways online. From the comfort of home, you can try gut-directed hypnotherapy by downloading an app to your smartphone. We like

Nerva, an app offering evidence-based hypnotherapy techniques designed to be used over a six-week period for fifteen minutes a day. Patients who complete the program see results comparable to results for those who complete treatment in person. Online group classes in gut-directed hypnosis have also been shown to be effective. See the Resources section for more digital-based therapeutics for IBS.

With hypnotherapy, a patient is guided safely and comfortably into a special mental state (hypnosis). What makes this form of relaxation training different from others is that it targets the subconscious mind. Typically we are unaware of the workings of the subconscious. By contrast, one is aware of what is going on in the conscious mind at a given moment, including thoughts and feelings. For example, on the one hand, you consciously think about your stomach problems, you consciously choose the words you speak about yourself or others, and you consciously try to avoid triggers for your IBS. Some refer to the conscious mind as the "doubting brain" because it can act with self-protective skepticism. On the other hand, the subconscious mind can be thought of as the psyche's gatekeeper. It contains all the information stored in your brain to manage your world, and it calls up that information only as needed. Without having to think about it, you are able to recall things (such as a memory from childhood, a phone number, how to construct a sentence, how to do math, etc.) and navigate life thanks to the subconscious. In hypnotherapy, the provider will verbally guide you into a deeply relaxed and highly focused state, which calms the conscious mind so that it plays a less active role in your thinking process.

During the hypnotic state, you remain aware of what is happening, but the conscious mind takes a rest. The subconscious mind becomes receptive to the gut-soothing and healing suggestions delivered during the hypnotherapy session. The suggestions are accompanied by peaceful imagery to illustrate and reinforce the desired therapeutic changes, which in IBS include improvements in gut function. For example, you might be asked to imagine your digestive tract as a stream and modify the flow of the water according to your needs—that is, decrease the flow if you have diarrhea or increase it if you have constipation. Additional treatment goals might include reducing the frequency and intensity of IBS distress, normalizing bowel activity, decreasing the reactivity of the GI tract to life stressors, and improving your overall physical quality of life. Hypnotherapy gets at the miscommunication between the brain and gut, and its ability to normalize central pain-processing patterns is impressive.

Although hypnosis may seem a bit unconventional, most people find the experience to be comfortable and even pleasurable. You may think that you are not someone who could be hypnotized. However, most people are hypnotizable to a degree. Have you ever spent your commute home daydreaming, arrived at home as though your car were on autopilot, and failed to remember much of the drive? That's like a hypnotic trance. During the session, don't fret if it seems that you're still "aware." Research has found that the depth of one's hypnotic state does not correlate with one's outcome to treatment. Furthermore, this intervention is safe, with no side effects. There is one exception: in the management of IBS, we do not recommend use of gut-directed hypnosis for those who are currently experiencing symptoms related to trauma. Because of the way you are learning how to deeply relax your body, if you have a trauma history, you should speak openly with your mental health provider about your comfort and emotions while doing mind-body work. In a clinical practice, a mental health provider will discuss whether hypnotherapy is recommended for you.

Finally, if you are struggling with anxiety and depression, prioritize that first. Gut-directed hypnotherapy, whether conducted in person, in a group, or via an app, is best received when mood symptoms are stable. If you would like to pursue gut-directed hypnotherapy in person, you can locate a trained expert in the Resources. You will want to ensure that the provider uses an evidence-based gut-directed hypnotherapy protocol, and that they are a licensed health professional.

After their first session, people who try hypnotherapy often comment, "I had no idea my body could be this relaxed." It provides a great deal of hope to people who have been suffering. They realize that they can in fact experience relief!

While we can't offer a full hypnotherapy treatment in this book, we do offer tips in this chapter for initiating relaxation on your own.

BRAIN BITE: CULTIVATE AN ACCEPTANCE MINDSET

Engaging in an acceptance mindset is critical to overall wellness. Let's take the weather as an example. You may have wanted to spend the day outside in the sun, but it is raining. You can stay indoors, angry about the rain, wishing it were different, and feeling your body tense up from frustration. Or you can accept that you can't change or control the weather. Come up with a new plan, or grab your umbrella and head out for a walk in the rain. Your acceptance mindset for handling challenges will translate into helpful skills when it comes to the management of IBS. Even the image of a warm walk in the rain (while metaphorically creating your own "sunshine" in your mind) may start you on your journey of using peaceful imagery to calm your body and mind.

SELF-GUIDED GUT-DIRECTED RELAXATION

In an earlier chapter, we introduced several ways you can meditate. Here we provide suggestions for a deeper, gut-directed relaxation practice. You will begin by deeply focusing your mind on relaxing the muscles of your body using a technique called passive muscle relaxation. Then you'll concentrate on soothing imagery (e.g., a peaceful place in nature) and on sensations intended to calm your IBS symptoms. Recent research has found that techniques utilizing metaphors and imagery—which strengthen one's inner resilience, enable self-compassion, and channel a mindset of acceptance—are incredibly helpful for managing stress. Mindfulness techniques, hypnosis, and other aspects of therapeutic work can all help you achieve this goal. So allow yourself the creative flexibility to use different techniques to create your own gut-directed relaxation practice.

We will get you started with a soothing practice that can help calm your mind and gut. You can ask a trusted friend or loved one to read this to you, record yourself reading it and replay as needed, or practice as you read the lines.

Let's Practice Gut-Directed Relaxation

Note that each of the three techniques outlined below can be used individually, but when used together they deepen the relaxation experience.

1. Focused Breathing with Passive Muscle Relaxation

Find a comfortable position. Settle into your space, finding comfort. Gently close your eyes when you are ready. Notice your breathing, and allow it to fall into a rhythm that feels slow and deep and regular. A comfortable rhythm for you. Pay attention to your breathing for about ten breaths.

Quietly shift your attention to the feelings in your body. Know that it is totally normal for your mind to wander. We call this the monkey mind. Sometimes it bounces into the future, which can create anxiety because things out there are unpredictable, uncontrollable. It's also very normal to find your mind wandering to the past, where things cannot be changed, which sometimes produces uncomfortable feelings. Bring your attention back to your breath if your mind floats too far. Again, these thoughts are completely normal, and as you settle into a mindful, relaxing practice, remind yourself that this is the time for calming your gut. Redirect your attention as needed, always bringing yourself back to the present moment, where you are allowed to relax your digestive system.

Notice the sensations in your hands. Allow your hands to lie open. Notice whether they feel warm or cool. Do they feel tense or relaxed? Heavy or light? Just allow your hands to lie wherever they are, becoming very comfortably relaxed, maybe a warmth and heaviness coming into them. Notice what that relaxation feels like in your palms and wrists. Feel the relaxation moving into your forearms. Your forearms are beginning to feel heavy. Comfortably relaxed. Move that sensation of relaxation into your upper arms, which begin to release stress and tension. Your arms gently begin to pull down from the shoulders, growing heavier and heavier. As this happens, the stress and tension that can so easily wind their way into your shoulders and upper back begin to fade away.

Release the weight on your shoulders. They are becoming more comfortable, loose, and relaxed. Think about something that you need to let go of, something that may rest heavily on your shoulders or your mind. Now is a good time to just release it, like you're untying a balloon and letting it drift away. The farther that stress-filled balloon floats away, the more relaxed your body becomes. You softly sink a little deeper into the state of focused relaxation. Maybe you need to let go of one more balloon before continuing, or maybe you're just beginning to enjoy the sensations of relaxation moving through your body. Your shoulders continue to be very relaxed, your neck is sharing in this relaxation, and you can let the relaxation move all the way up to the top of your head.

The muscles in your forehead are unwinding and loosening. Those muscles may feel almost like rubber bands that are tightly knotted. Now, with a nice, gentle exhalation, release any stress and tension. The rubber bands are unwinding, leaving you with a calm, clear mind. Let the relaxation move through the muscles of your face, smoothing out the areas around your eyes, cheeks, and jaw. You are becoming more and more relaxed. Maybe you found tension in your jaw. Let your teeth part slightly as your jaw hangs like a hinge.

Your breathing is very slow, deep, and regular. During this practice, you may find that you need to move your muscles around to release and relax them. Maybe now you notice that it would feel good to pull your shoulders up toward your ears, feel the tension, and then let them go again, allowing them to drop back down as far away from the ears as they can. You are sinking into a very comfortable state of relaxation. Your shoulders are comfortably relaxed, and you feel the relaxation moving downward, loosening the muscles of your upper back. You also feel a soothing sensation moving into your chest.

Your stomach is becoming calm. You are breathing freely and slowly and deeply. Notice if your heartbeat has found a slow and relaxed rhythm. Your stomach is beginning to share in this comfortable sensation, becoming deeply relaxed. And now the lower part of your body begins to relax. Your lower back, your hips, and your thighs are becoming heavy, heavy, and very relaxed.

Your legs and feet get heavier. You sink further into this safe, comfortable space, noticing that your legs begin to share in the deep, heavy, warm relaxation. Your legs become heavier as they grow deeply relaxed, all the way down into your feet. Your feet are heavy and relaxed. Notice a warmth throughout your feet all the way into your toes.

2. Cloud Deepening into a Focused, Relaxed State

Your body is now deeply relaxed. As your relaxation deepens, begin to envision yourself sitting or lying on a supersoft, bouncy cloud. Imagine that it is holding you very securely, in the most comfortable and soothing way, as you float into a state of calm, deep relaxation. We will begin to count from one to twenty, and with each number the cloud will gently carry you deeper into a state of focused relaxation.

1 . . . You sink deeply into this comfortable and relaxing state. . . .

2 . . . A state where you become very focused on allowing your entire mind and body to be at ease . . .

3 . . . 4 . . . There is nothing to bother you right now. . . .

5 . . . 6 . . . 7 . . . There is nothing else to worry about and no other place to be right now. This is your time for deep relaxation . . .

8 . . . 9 . . . 10 . . . The cloud continues to carry you down into a deep, safe, very comfortable state of relaxation . . .

11 . . . 12 . . . 13 . . . 14 . . . In this state, your mind is focused on allowing your body deep peace and relaxation . . .

15 . . . You're descending into a deep, focused state where your stomach and intestines share in the deep relaxation of your other muscles . . .

16 . . . Deeper and deeper . . .

17 . . . 18 . . . Your mind and your body relaxing even more . . .

19 . . . 20 . . . You are now in a very deep and focused state of comfortable relaxation.

3. Gut-Directed Guided Imagery for Relaxation

Picture a beautiful place. With your body and your mind more and more relaxed, you begin to focus your attention on an image of a very safe and beautiful place in nature. A comfortable place that you know well and where you feel safe and welcome. Perhaps it is a place you have been many times, or maybe your mind takes you to an imaginary place. Wherever this tranquil place is, you feel at ease and at peace, and your body continues to relax very deeply.

Imagine sitting down in a comfortable chair. You are still in the glorious place in nature and beginning to take in all the beauty around you. Perhaps you feel the sun shining down, warming your skin. You may also notice a gentle breeze that works with the sun to create the most perfectly comfortable temperature for you. A gentle warmth begins to move through you, bringing a soothing sensation of relaxation that permeates your entire body. This comfortable, gentle warmth soothes the stomach and intestines in a way that feels healing and relieving to your digestive tract.

Allow yourself to experience this place with all your available senses. You continue to look around you. What else do you see? What do you hear? Perhaps you hear a gentle wind moving the leaves of tall trees around you. Or maybe you are near water, and you hear the peaceful sound of a creek flowing or waves softly rolling in on a shore. Maybe you notice a comforting fragrance.

Bring the comfort of this place to your stomach and your intestines. This peaceful place becomes more vivid and clear to you. Allow the same comfort that your senses are experiencing to bring comfort and peace to your stomach and intestines. As your body and mind continue to relax, you also relax more deeply inside your body. Feel this relaxation spreading through your entire digestive tract, filling your stomach and intestines with a soothing warmth that brings a confidence in your ability to feel comfort. With this deep relaxation spreading throughout your body, your bowels are becoming less and less sensitive to stress.

You feel only comfort. In this very peaceful place, perhaps you feel that you are only able to experience deep peace and pleasant sensations. You will not allow any discomfort or pain to bother you right now. And you are beginning to build confidence in your ability to maintain a deep, soothing state of comfort inside your digestive tract no matter what stress you are faced with. Each time you allow yourself to experience deep relaxation inside, your body improves its ability to maintain that soothing comfort from day to day. Allow yourself a few moments now to deepen the relaxation you feel throughout your whole body as you continue to experience your tranquil place. Allow yourself to become more and more relaxed. Allow your whole body to sink deeper into this carefree state of comfort. Focus on the ability of your mind to heal and soothe your entire digestive tract.

Allow two minutes of quiet and calm.

Slowly come back to the present. It is time to envision yourself slowly standing up from your chair in this tranquil place. Begin to allow your tranquil place to dissolve gradually from your mind as you return. (But you can allow yourself to return to this comfortable, familiar, peaceful place whenever your body or mind needs to, whenever you need a few moments of calm.) Slowly begin to count backward from 20 to 1. On the count of 1 your eyes will open, and you will return to your day feeling refreshed and calm. Your digestive tract will also be refreshed and calm. When your eyes open, you will have no uncomfortable aftereffects; you will only feel at ease and at peace.

20 . . . 19 . . . Slowly beginning to bring yourself back to awareness . . .

18 . . . 17 . . . 16 . . . 15 . . . 14 . . . 13 . . . 12 . . . 11 . . . 10 . . . Becoming more alert . . .

9 . . . 8 . . . 7 . . . 6 . . . 5 . . . Closer to opening your eyes . . .

4 . . . 3 . . . 2 . . . and . . . 1 . . . Your eyes open. You are relaxed and completely alert.

AUTOGENIC TRAINING

Autogenic training is a self-induced relaxation technique that can be thought of as self-hypnosis to promote feelings of calm and relaxation in the body. It focuses on six areas of the body and mind. For each area, you will repeat to yourself several different sentences in a specific pattern: silently repeat the designated sentence, then close your eyes and repeat the sentence five more times before moving on to the next one. Set a pace that is slow, relaxed, and comfortable. Take about five seconds to say each sentence, and allow a three-second pause between each repetition to focus on what you have said. If you don't internally *feel* what you are saying, repeat it a couple more times. Feeling the heaviness and warmth may take some time, so keep practicing. Feel free to adjust the phrases to find what is most comfortable for you.

Let's Practice Autogenics

Find a safe, comfortable place, and settle in. For each of the statements written below, proceeding one sentence at a time, say it slowly to yourself once, then close your eyes and repeat it five more times.

Focus on heaviness. "My right arm is heavy. My left arm is heavy. Both my arms are heavy. My right leg is heavy. My left leg is heavy. Both my legs are heavy. My arms and my legs are heavy."

Focus on warmth. "My right arm is warm. My left arm is warm. Both my arms are warm. My left leg is warm. My right leg is warm. Both my legs are warm. My arms and my legs are warm."

Focus on a calm heartbeat. "My arms are heavy and warm. My legs are heavy and warm. My arms and legs are heavy and warm. I feel calm. My heart feels warm and at peace. My heartbeat is calm and steady."

Focus on breathing. "My arms are heavy and warm. My legs are heavy and warm. My arms and legs are heavy and warm. I feel calm. My heartbeat is calm and steady. My breathing is deep and soothing."

Focus on soothing the stomach. "My arms are heavy and warm. My legs are heavy and warm. I feel calm. My heart feels calm. My heartbeat is steady. My breathing is deep and regular. My stomach is soft, warm, and at ease."

Focus on a cool forehead. "My arms are heavy and warm. My legs are heavy and warm. My arms and my legs are heavy and warm. I feel calm. My heartbeat is calm and steady. My breathing is deep and regular. My stomach is soft, warm, and at ease. My forehead is calm and cool."

Complete this practice by stating an intention, following the same pattern as above: one time with eyes open, and five more times with eyes closed. For example, "My body and mind are completely calm. I am so capable of managing my health."

GUT GAME CHANGER:
THE I LOVE YOU MASSAGE

This is an abdominal massage technique that can help move stool and gas through your colon, which may relieve uncomfortable cramping, bloating, pressure, and tightness. You will use your fingers to make patterns in the shape of the letters I, L, and U (hence the name).

1. Lie down on the floor or on a firm mattress.
2. Place both hands on the left side of your abdomen, below the ribs. Using light pressure, make small circles with your fingertips, moving in a straight line down toward your left hip. (This is the I pattern.)
3. Next, still making small circles, run your fingertips from the right side of your upper abdomen down along the ribs and across the bottom of the ribs toward the left side (the L pattern).
4. Now start at the bottom right side of your abdomen, near the hip, and make small circles up the right side, across the lower ribs, and down the left side, creating a U pattern.

Disclaimer: This technique does not replace medical advice from your health-care provider. Talk to your health-care provider if you have any questions about this technique.

Living with IBS, you may have been at odds with your body. As you begin to connect with your body and regularly practice relaxation interventions, you will notice changes in the way you cope with your IBS symptoms. You'll improve the relationship you have with your body and reap the emotional benefits of healthy healing as well.

MOVE YOUR BODY, SOOTHE YOUR GUT

Up to this point, you've been establishing a relaxation routine that involves being still. In that stillness you are learning to be with your body in a way that releases stress and tension, which is helpful for your digestive health. But it is also important to get moving. No matter the type of IBS you experience, a consistent exercise routine can help. In times of stress, the neuroendocrine response produces chemicals, such as adrenaline, that can worsen IBS. Physical activity can counteract those effects and positively affect brain plasticity. That is, the brain can actually rewire itself as a result of engaging in new, healthy behaviors. Exercise can also help protect against worsening IBS symptoms. Increasing your physical activity can change gas transit and colonic transit, which can contribute to symptom improvement.

We are all individuals with different abilities and interests when it comes to moving our bodies. Some have disabilities, activity limitations, or participation restrictions that inform the way they engage in movement. It is important to listen to your body and make modifications as needed. If exercise is not a regular part of your week, you can change that! You just need to find an activity that brings you joy. Begin with chair-based yoga, gentle stretching, or walking, or put on some music and dance in your living room. Researchers have shown that any form of moderate physical activity—engaged in three times a week for periods ranging from twenty to sixty minutes—can improve the severity of IBS symptoms. If that sounds like a lot, start with baby steps, then add more activity. If you want to exercise in the comfort of your home initially, check out home yoga videos to get you started. (See the Resources section for some inspiration.)

Research also shows the importance of consistency in your exercise routine. After four months of consistent, moderate physical activity, our patients have seen sustained positive effects not only on their IBS symptoms but also on their quality of life, fatigue, anxiety, and other mood symptoms.

So many types of exercise programs exist these days that you will surely be able to find one that works for you and that you enjoy. The answer to the question "What type of exercise should I do?" is "Whichever one you like and will stick with." Below, we highlight two forms of movement that most people can engage in: walking and yoga. They are simple, and they complement each other well. (Special note: If you are someone who trains intensively, such as an elite athlete or ultramarathoner, be aware of the potential negative effects of too much exercise on gut symptoms. You may need to consult a physician to discuss how your exercise regimen could be affecting your IBS.)

Walking gets the blood flowing, lubricates the joints to improve mobility, builds strength throughout the body, increases energy, improves balance and coordination, and enhances cardiovascular fitness and bone health. When you are walking for aerobic exercise, you want to set yourself up for success by setting goals that are achievable and safe. If you aren't yet in a routine, begin with committing to a ten-minute walk each day until it becomes a habit. Just as we have suggested scheduling time for relaxation, schedule time for your exercise. "I will take a ten-minute walk during my lunch period." "I will take a twenty-minute walk after work." "Our family will walk for twenty minutes after dinner." Consider exercising with a partner to help create accountability. Find what works for you, make it enjoyable, and keep it consistent.

Also, if you miss a day, remember that you are human! Perhaps your body was telling you it needed a day of rest. Remind yourself of your goals and of the benefits you are experiencing, and get back on track the following day.

Yoga can beautifully combine the principles of focused aware-ness and body movement. Many different styles exist. The most common techniques focus on body postures (asanas), breathing (pra-nayama), and meditation (dhyana). Yoga instructors often combine several methods tailored to a specific class. Yoga to soothe the gut typically involves easy breathing practices, abdominal stretching, twisting postures, and resting the body. While more robust research into the specific benefits of yoga for people with IBS is needed, a review of the literature indicates it is a safe adjunctive (nonessen-tial) treatment. Yoga appears to be beneficial for stress reduction and alteration of the brain-gut interaction. It also may help promote pos-itive changes to the gut microbiome in those who are concurrently making dietary changes.

Here are some tips for developing a gut-friendly yoga practice:

- If you are a beginner yogi, we recommend attending at least a couple of classes in person. Almost all beginner classes will introduce you to skills that you can practice at your own pace and comfort level.
- Try different instructors, studios, or types of yoga to find a practice you enjoy. (Some of our favorite online programs for yoga and other exercises to promote healthy digestion are listed in the Resources.)
- Modifications for various poses are usually provided throughout a class. You are encouraged to meet yourself where you are. It's also important to develop the skill of hon-oring your body during a class by pausing, taking a break, and choosing rest when needed.

- As your skills and excitement for yoga grow, you may find it beneficial to practice at home some of the poses you learn in class.

SELF-AFFIRMATIONS FOR MANAGING YOUR HEALTH

A yoga practice sometimes ends with an affirmation. Again, your internal dialogue influences how you feel physically and emotionally. Healing while living with IBS requires developing a kind inner voice. Sometimes discomfort in the body serves as a sign that it's time to regulate thoughts and emotions and bring the body back to a calm state—that's where CBT comes in. As you catch your thoughts, you can check them and change them (the three Cs). You can also use the power of self-affirmation.

The science of self-affirmation is real! A large review of the literature showed that correct use of self-affirmation has many benefits. It can decrease stress, increase well-being, make people more open to behavioral changes, improve academic performance, and assist in coping with situations that present threat.

Self-affirmations are defined as acts that acknowledge one's self-worth. To create a self-affirmation, a key is to reflect on your personal core values and your broader sense of self. For example, you are far more than someone who is navigating IBS day-to-day; you may be a loving parent, a thoughtful partner, a helpful neighbor, a genuine friend, a trusted employee. When you are faced with life's stressors, you can use this knowledge to move beyond them by focusing on your competence and worth. Affirmations help people maintain a narrative of personal adequacy in difficult circumstances—"I can handle this!" Using them can make you more resilient. You are using healthy coping skills instead of falling back into unhelpful stress responses.

Recite your self-affirmations at the beginning of your day, during a stressful moment, or before going to sleep at night. You can also teach your loved ones about the power of a good self-affirmation. A child who knows their self-worth has a good foundation for becoming a healthy adult, so spread these skills widely! Before we identify affirmations that might work for you, let's explore the core values that lie at the heart of believable affirmations.

DISCOVER YOUR CORE VALUES

Your personal core values offer guiding principles for your life in terms of how you carry yourself around others (or when others are not around), when setting goals, and when making decisions. They are what you view as ideal standards for living—for instance, being kind and honest. We often develop core values based on the people who were around us during our childhood. Parents or caregivers, extended family members, friends, teachers, religious leaders, community—all factor into the development of core values.

While some of your core values may remain consistent throughout your life, such as valuing education and hard work, you may experience shifts in your values or add new ones. For example, maybe fitness or health were not big focuses for you until someone invited you to a yoga class. After attending classes for a few months, maybe you found yourself committed to weekly classes, finding joy and connection in your yoga community and benefiting far beyond the physical aspects of your practice. You now place strong value in your health, which helps generate energy and vitality that affect your overall well-being. As you integrate aspects of health, nutrition, time for self-care, and improvements in coping skills, you may see other positive additions to your core values.

Use the list provided in Table 8 to identify your current core values. Remember that you can aspire to add to your list.

TABLE 8. CORE VALUES

Health	Patience	Learning	Purpose
Collaboration	Acceptance	Strength	Balance
Creativity	Compassion	Courage	Respect
Family	Love	Mindfulness	Hard work
Independence	Curiosity	Enjoyment	Fairness
Kindness	Togetherness	Spirituality	Responsibility
Leadership	Intelligence	Peace	Principle
Skillfulness	Stability	Achievement	Resilience
Competence	Adventure	Wealth	Humor
Integrity	Energy	Success	Consistency

WHAT ARE YOUR CORE VALUES?

Now that you have spent time identifying your core values, you are ready to create your self-affirmations. These, too, may change over time, but let's focus on affirmations that will be most powerful to you today. Using a broad self-affirmation, such as "I am awesome," is not the goal here. These types of generic affirmations are not effective when you don't believe you are awesome at this moment. The goal is to come up with statements that accurately and authentically connect with your personal truth. You can also choose statements that highlight your evolving journey and what you want to eventually believe. For example, *I am working every day to improve my health. I am becoming capable of facing challenging situations with my IBS. I am trying each day to think more positively about myself.*

We have listed examples of self-affirmations for wellness that we find useful, but we encourage you to take time to review your list of core values and use them to create a few self-affirmations of your own.

Five Daily Affirmations for Wellness

1. Exactly as I am, I am good enough and I am valued.
2. Every day I am becoming healthier.
3. I am supported and loved during the process of healing.
4. My body is powerful and capable.
5. I deserve to take time for myself.

My Personal Affirmations

1. _____

2. _____

3. _____

4. _____

5. _____

There is incredible power in knowing your worth. *You deserve good health and a full life.* As you begin to prioritize spending time to help your body and mind relax, your mindset around how you approach the various demands of life will change for the better. As this chapter has shown, you have tools available to diminish the effects of stress. You can engage in a gut-directed relaxation practice, hit the road for a walk, or take to the mat for a yoga class. With a better handle on your relaxation response, you can take on life's challenges and joys with more energy and optimism.

CHAPTER 5

NUTRITIONAL REMEDIES TO CALM AND SOOTHE YOUR IBS GUT

"Can I eat that?" When eating food seems to commonly trigger digestive distress, it's no wonder you are not sure what to eat. We get that and are ready to arm you with nutritional tools backed by science. Whether you are prone to diarrhea or constipation, or experience bloating, your diet should be tailored to you and your gut symptoms. As with most things related to IBS, a one-size diet does not fit all. In this chapter, we'll provide you with a better understanding of how certain foods may be players in your GI distress and step-by-step ways to adapt your diet. Strategies that work for you may include reducing your intake of poorly digested carbohydrates (e.g., FODMAPs), changing your fiber intake, or adjusting when and how you eat.

Of course, working with a dietitian is the ideal way to help you sort out your food triggers and design a dietary intervention suitable for your lifestyle, budget, and health goals. A list of web-sites in the Resources (see page 327) can help you find one. But we also realize that not everyone has access to a GI-expert dietitian due to insurance coverage or geographical location. With that in mind, to kick-start you in the right direction, the next few chapters offer comprehensive guidance on the many ways that food plays a role in IBS.

No matter what, we want you eating the widest variety of foods you can tolerate. Well-balanced and nutritious eating is a goal for all of us. When selecting the best nutritional path for managing your IBS symptoms, you (and your dietitian, if you have one) should always focus on the most liberal and nourishing food plan possible. Less is not more when it comes to good nutrition. For some people with IBS, our gentle diet cleanup plan may be the best route to go rather than following a limited diet. For those who have severe IBS symptoms, a more restrictive diet, such as a low-FODMAP elimi-nation diet, may indeed be indicated to quell the gut. As you navi-gate your IBS treatments, this book will arm you with a plethora of options you can select in conjunction with your health-care team to best fit your needs. Together, you can discuss the pros and cons of various diets to find the one that is the best choice for you.

ARE DIET CHANGES RIGHT FOR YOU?

Most people living with IBS want to try diet therapies to help man-age their gut symptoms. Sometimes this is rooted in a desire to have some control over their health due to the lack of control one can feel when struggling with IBS. We get it! Although diet can be a healthy and powerful intervention for IBS, it sometimes comes with cave-ats. Before you begin tinkering with what you eat, it's vital to make sure that a dietary intervention is appropriate for you. Alternative approaches might be a greater priority if:

- You have a history of an eating disorder.
- You have already severely restricted your diet without symptom improvement.
- You are struggling to add foods back to your diet.
- You find that stress is the factor that most regularly affects your symptoms.

For some people, becoming too focused on diet leads to over-restriction of foods and an inability to enjoy the social aspects of eating, which in turn can lead to a slippery slope of disordered eating. Disordered eating patterns occur when someone skips meals, limits many foods or food groups, or follows a restrictive diet *beyond* what is deemed medically appropriate to avoid or prevent symptoms. Scientific studies reveal that people living with health conditions that require a special diet as part of the treatment—such as diabetes, celiac disease, inflammatory bowel disease, and IBS—run a higher risk of disordered eating.

We also know that individuals with a history of eating disorders (such as anorexia nervosa, a condition associated with extreme food restriction and fear of weight gain) have a higher likelihood of developing IBS, an effect that is thought to be due to the negative impact of malnutrition on the gut and the gut microbes. We examine disordered eating (including orthorexia, which is characterized by an obsession with healthy eating) in greater detail in Chapter 7 and provide resources for guidance with eating disorders in the Resources section.

WHEN DIET *IS* A GOOD TREATMENT CHOICE

With all that said, making diet changes might be right for you if:

- Eating triggers GI symptoms.

Why: If eating does not lead to your digestive symptoms, then it is unlikely food is your IBS symptom trigger.

- You do not have a history of an eating disorder or do not experience severe anxiety or extreme fear associated with food or eating.

  Why: Most diet therapies for IBS involve elimination of foods. In an individual with an eating disorder history or significant anxiety associated with food or eating, eliminating foods could retrigger or further add to the food-fear experiences, increasing the risk of maladaptive eating or potentially an eating disorder.

- You have been recently screened for celiac disease.

  Why: A gluten-free or low-FODMAP diet reduces gluten intake, and one must be consuming gluten for the test for celiac disease to be accurate. Before you remove gluten from your diet, make sure you first get checked for celiac disease in case that is the root cause of your symptoms.

- You are interested in changing your diet and have the means (i.e., the cooking ability and finances) to follow a specific diet.

  Why: In a motivated patient, diet change can be very successful in managing IBS symptoms. Research has shown that people with numerous food intolerances are more likely to have severe IBS and a poorer quality of life (QOL). Diet change can be validating and empowering while improving QOL along with gut symptoms.

A RELAY RACE TO SUCCESS

Finding *your* best diet for IBS can be compared to taking part in a relay race. Each runner uniquely provides their own contribution to winning the race, and they each do so in their own way. As you lace up, remember that your nutritional needs differ from other people's, and navigating what works for *you* is how your race will unfold. You are working toward your own personal record. You and your health-care team can establish your individual benchmark by which to measure your success. And remember, success can be found through improved confidence in using your coping skills to calm symptoms, which leads to less anxiety as well as less frequent and less severe flare-ups.

DIGESTIBLE DETAIL: HOW DO I KNOW MY DIET ADJUSTMENT IS WORKING?

- Your digestive symptoms are improving.
- You are able to dine out with friends and family.
- The food you eat brings you great pleasure.
- You can still incorporate some of your favorite foods.
- You can easily meet your nutritional needs.
- Your dietary changes have allowed you to travel more and have a fuller life.
- You are not constantly thinking about food.

Because each IBS body has its own fingerprint of gut microbes and its very particular set of symptoms, some people simply need a dietary "cleanup"—for example, making changes to reduce common GI triggers (fat, alcohol, caffeine), or adding food components, such as certain fibers to bulk up or soften the stool. Others may need a bigger diet overhaul, such as incorporating the low-FODMAP elimination diet. Figuring this out can be a bit of a process—and that's okay. We'll say it once again for those in the back of the room: the least restrictive diet that offers symptom management is always the goal. For overall quality of life and to establish a good relationship with food, your personal best is what matters.

THE GENTLE DIET CLEANUP (AKA START HERE!)

For the initial step, we recommend giving your dietary routine a good once-over to see if common GI triggers or eating habits are playing a role in your digestive symptoms. For instance, overindulgence in caffeinated beverages, fatty foods, spicy foods, or alcohol can prompt GI distress in anyone, never mind the potential impact on someone with a sensitive gut. Try the following general modifications in diet and lifestyle before moving on to any elimination diet such as the low-FODMAP diet (outlined later in the chapter).

As with any science-based intervention, it's best to try one approach or dietary change at a time to be able to discern what is working or, alternatively, what may be making symptoms worse. Generally speaking, most treatments should be trialed for up to a month or six weeks max. Treatments that do not offer symptom relief after you give them a fair trial should be discontinued with the guidance of your health-care provider.

Our gentle diet cleanup plan encourages dialing back on some of the most common scientifically recognized IBS triggers. It's based on many of the key concepts of the United Kingdom's (UK's) National Institute for Health and Care Excellence (NICE) guidelines for IBS care, and also incorporates other adjustments. Here are the strategies:

- Eat at regular times (three meals per day and a snack or two).
- Take time to eat (a meal should last longer than fifteen minutes).

- Chew food completely. Digestion starts in your mouth!
- Ensure that you are in a comfortable eating environment and in a relaxed state for the best digestion at mealtimes.
- Avoid skipping meals.
- Drink eight cups of fluid per day, primarily water.
- Restrict caffeinated coffee and tea to three cups per day.
- Reduce alcohol and carbonated drinks (one alcoholic drink per day maximum for women, two drinks for men; carbonated drinks based on your tolerance).
- Limit foods rich in insoluble fiber (whole wheat breads, wheat-bran-based cereals), based on your tolerance.
- Limit fresh fruit to three servings per day.
- If constipation is present, try to incorporate two medium-sized green kiwifruit (equates to one fruit serving) per day or on most days.
- If experiencing diarrhea, reduce sorbitol-containing foods and products (sorbitol is found in sugar-free gum, sugar-free mints, stone fruits, and prunes).
- Minimize high-fat meals—goodbye, fried food platters!
- Reduce overly spicy foods (e.g., chili peppers, extra spicy Thai or Indian food, hot sauces).

One recent study from the UK comparing the traditional NICE IBS guidelines to a low-FODMAP and gluten-free diet found that all three diets offered good IBS symptom control. The NICE guidelines, however, offered a few extra lifestyle benefits: the diet required less time to shop for and was easier to follow when eating out with family and friends.

Let's get into some of the main principles of the cleanup approach, along with the details about why certain things may get your tummy in a bunch—for example, meal size, skipping meals, too much fat, certain fibers, hot spices, and caffeine or alcohol overload.

1. Meal Timing and Size Matter: Don't Skip Meals!

Eating at regular times is a key feature of the gentle diet cleanup. It's not uncommon for individuals living with IBS to avoid eating during the day in an effort to minimize GI distress while out and about or at work. Sorry, but this strategy generally backfires. Here's the deal. We all need to eat at regular intervals to fuel our body and mind. From a young age, our body needs three meals (and, often, two snacks) per day to give us enough energy to meet our physical and mental demands. Eating about every three to four hours sets the stage for good health and a good mood. When we ignore the body's hunger messages, our blood sugar can plummet and lead to other hormonal imbalances. You know the feeling—getting cranky, irritable, *hangry*.

If you skip meals, the body will try to make up the calories and energy the next time food is readily available. This potentially sets up the cycle of "bingeing" on food in the evening. Eating a huge amount of food at once is a lot for the gut to process. It can lead to poor absorption of food and then GI distress while you're trying to sleep or as you awaken. Having GI symptoms in the morning can prompt the cycle of restriction and overeating again. This starve-binge cycle ultimately doesn't work out well for a sensitive gut.

Eating three meals a day is a gentler nutrition therapy for improved absorption of food in the gut and less digestive distress.

As you learn your IBS food triggers (we'll get into those), soon you will be able to identify what foods work in your belly—and what foods do not. When you trust your food, you can relax when you eat. Remember that gut and brain are linked. When you are feeling relaxed, you are able to digest food more effectively and efficiently. Keeping food portions reasonable and balanced during the day is your best plan for better digestion.

Keep in mind that if skipping breakfast or lunch has been normal for you, adapting to a more structured eating pattern may lead to some initial, albeit short-lived, pushback from your gut. It may take a couple of weeks for your body (and the microbes that reside in your gut) to adapt to your new eating pattern. If you experience extra bloating or cramping with your diet change, consider implementing some of the special breathing and relaxation techniques outlined in Chapters 2, 3, and 4. These strategies will help ease your transition. Remember, a runner will not achieve their personal record without good nutrition to fuel the run. Success comes from the structured practice and coaching (from your health-care team) that guides your way.

The bottom line: Don't skip meals, relax when eating, chew your food well (this allows the digestive enzymes in your mouth to start working), eat three meals per day (made up of foods that you tolerate), and, depending on your hunger level, enjoy a snack or two.

BRAIN BITE: BREAKFAST, WELCOME BACK!

You may not feel hungry in the morning if you have been skipping breakfast for years. However, changing this behavior and reintroducing breakfast to your routine will have long-term benefits. Start your day with the intention to fuel your body and your mind, eat a nutritious breakfast, and soothe your gut with a couple of minutes of diaphragmatic breathing. Congratulations—you have just fueled your day with some really positive vibes!

Another reason to eat breakfast: Eating stimulates the gastrocolic reflex, which signals to the colon that it's time to have a bowel movement. For people prone to constipation, eating breakfast is super important, as it preps the body for a morning poop.

2. Hydrate, Hydrate, Hydrate

Your body is about 55 to 60 percent water, and your brain is 70 percent water. That's a lot! To stay healthy, it's important to replenish the fluids that you lose via respiration, sweat, urine, and stool. If you're prone to diarrhea, consuming even more fluids is vital for keeping hydrated so that your body can properly perform other bodily functions. Water is also critical for proper digestion; it can work with the fiber in food to help normalize bowel movements.

The bottom line: Do your best to get in your eight 8-ounce glasses of water per day, particularly if you are prone to diarrhea or live an active (sweaty) lifestyle. Fill a glass pitcher with 64 ounces of water, and try to finish it before the end of the day. You can also keep yourself accountable in terms of your water consumption for a week or two by using the Mind Your Gut Food and Lifestyle Tracker, found in the Resources.

3. Consider All Those Cups of Coffee

Let's start with the good news: a little coffee can be good for you. Coffee is a key source of many bioactive compounds that offer health benefits. Interestingly, consuming three cups of coffee per day is associated with living a long life and lowering the risk of all-cause mortality. The bad news: while coffee may offer surprising benefits, it first meets our body via—you guessed it—the GI tract and can lead to heartburn and diarrhea in some people.

The morning cup of joe is well known for prompting a trip to the loo. About 30 percent of people notice that coffee makes them poop. It appears to affect lower colonic function by enhancing motor responses, which moves the intestinal contents to prepare the body to poop. Coffee stimulates the release of gastrin (from the stomach), which increases colonic movements, and cholecystokinin (from the small intestine), which releases bile and digestive enzymes, initiating the digestive process. Women tend to be more sensitive to the rectal distention associated with coffee's effects (and more likely to be diagnosed with IBS).

If you have IBS with a constipation predominance, a little stimulation to the gut via coffee may help with better bowel movement regularity, whereas if you have diarrhea predominance, you may find that less caffeine is a better plan. Keep in mind that caffeine is not just found in coffee. It is found in chocolate, tea, many sodas, and energy and sports drinks. Also, not all "cups" are created equal. See Table 9 for the caffeine content of common drinks.

TABLE 9. CAFFEINE CONTENT OF COMMON BEVERAGES

Food/beverage	Serving size	Amount of caffeine (approximate)
Coffee	8 ounces, brewed	95 mg
Black tea	8 ounces	47 mg
Green tea	8 ounces	25 mg
Chocolate milk	8 ounces	2 mg
Cola	8 ounces	24 mg

The bottom line: Drinking coffee might help or hinder your IBS depending on whether you are prone to diarrhea or constipation. Either way, though, know your caffeine limits. Consume no more than 24 ounces of coffee per day, or the equivalent of about 300 milligrams (mg) caffeine from any beverages or food, particularly if you have IBS-D.

DIGESTIBLE DETAIL: WHAT'S IN YOUR COFFEE?

Although you may think the trigger to your gut symptoms is the caffeine in your morning cup of liquid energy, it might be what you are adding to it. Extra sugar, sugar-free sweeteners, FODMAP-containing milks such as most soy milks, extra cream (fat), or extra milk (lactose) can exacerbate your gut symptoms too. The brand of coffee and style of preparation (drip, pour-over, cold brew, etc.) can also affect the caffeine content of your coffee.

4. Minimize Bubbles and Booze

Bubbly and fizzy drinks are fun to sip but maybe not so fun for your belly. Carbonated beverages such as soft drinks, seltzer, beer, and champagne can trigger bloating, heartburn, or indigestion for some people with IBS. If you find that the gas in your beverages exacerbates your tummy woes, try sticking with still beverages instead.

Drinking too much alcohol can also cause GI symptoms. A moderate amount of alcohol (one drink or less per day for women; two drinks or less for men) does not appear to be a symptom trigger in IBS. A glass of wine to toast the weekend should be tolerated by most people living with IBS. Cheers to that! But binge drinking (consuming four or more drinks on a single occasion) is another story. Binge drinking is associated with GI symptoms, particularly diarrhea, nausea, stomach pain, and indigestion, in individuals with IBS-D. Chronic excessive alcohol intake can alter GI motility, damage the gut lining (leading to intestinal permeability, or leakiness), affect nutrient absorption, and lead to intestinal inflammation. Moreover, excessive alcohol consumption can change the gut microbiota and is associated with elevated bacterial endotoxin levels, which in turn are associated with increased gut permeability.

Take inventory of your alcohol consumption. How much are you drinking per week? It might be more than you think. Look at the Gut Game Changer sidebar below and calculate your weekly intake by actual serving size. Women should consume no more than seven drinks per week, and men should limit to fourteen or less. Truthfully, less is more when it comes to alcohol, as consumption is linked with increased risk of cancer of the rectum, colon, liver, and esophagus.

GUT GAME CHANGER: WHAT IS ONE DRINK ANYWAY?

Know your limits for better gut health:

A serving of alcohol for a woman = one drink/day

A serving of alcohol for a man = two drinks/day

1 serving of beer = 12 ounces (5 percent alcohol)

1 serving of wine = 5 ounces (12 percent alcohol)

1 serving of spirits = 1.5 ounces (40 percent alcohol/80 proof)

Be mindful also that drinking alcohol may result in letting your guard down, causing you to veer into food-trigger territory when you drink. The combo of snack foods and alcohol may be an added irritant to your gut.

The bottom line: Alcohol is a potential gut irritant and can contribute to GI distress. Know your limits, and dial back on the booze if you are consuming too much. Limiting carbonated beverages may help reduce gas in the gut, minimizing bloating sensations.

5. Don't Chew Too Much Fat

Fatty foods (think greasy burger and fries, pizza, even extra cream in your morning coffee) have been identified by people living with IBS as prime food triggers. They can lead to increased gas, bloating, distention, and diarrhea. In fact, two survey studies found that IBS patients connected the dots between their fat intake and digestive distress.

Fatty foods have been shown to increase gut hypersensitivity and delay the GI transit of gas. Another problem tends to be the large portions that are often served at restaurants, which can up a person's overall fat intake to flare levels. A small handful of french fries probably won't contain enough fat to set your gut off, but when you "supersize that order," there may be a price to pay.

So what can you do? Spreading your intake of dietary fat throughout the day may help with tolerance. And there are plenty of healthy fats you can eat. We actually recommend a dose of healthy fat (found in nuts, seeds, nut butters, extra-virgin olive oil, avocado, salmon) at every meal, as these foods offer benefits for the heart and gut (by feeding the good bacteria) and can keep your body feeling pleasantly satiated—full but not too full. Healthy fats often offer polyphenols, a source of prebiotics that foster the growth of health-promoting gut microbes. We recommend nuts and seeds in particular as great sources of plant protein, fiber, vitamins, and minerals.

The bottom line: Go easy on fried foods—or limit them to special occasions. Select healthy fat options, and enjoy them spread out throughout the day for better tolerance. Opt for lower-fat meal-prep methods, such as baking, grilling, or broiling. Start incorporating healthy fats by snacking on a handful of nuts or seeds, adding a few slices of avocado to a salad or sandwich, enjoying a grilled salmon steak, or drizzling extra-virgin olive oil over roasted veggies or a mixed green salad.

6. Make Friends with Fiber

Fiber is the indigestible part of plant foods, and it is found in fruits, vegetables, legumes (beans and peas), nuts, seeds, and whole grains. Humans lack the digestive enzymes necessary to break down fiber for digestion and absorption in the small intestine, and that is where our colonic gut microbes come in.

Our colon is a living petri dish, containing about 70 percent of all the microbes that reside in our body. Our gut microbes, or flora, stay busy eating what escapes digestion in the small intestine. Most of the gut flora contains digestive enzymes capable of breaking down fiber. One type of gut microbe may start the process, and another type will swoop in and finish the job. When they consume fiber, they can create copious gas and numerous metabolites (substances created by the microbes and used by the body). No two humans' microbiomes are alike, so we all have our own bacterial responses to consumption of fiber. This presents a unique IBS challenge.

Although a fiber-rich diet is generally associated with many positive health outcomes—including lowering risk of colon cancer, reducing cholesterol, managing blood sugar, and helping maintain the protective gut barrier—we are learning that with IBS, there is more to the story. Each person's tolerance of different fibers can vary.

Fiber comes in many shapes and forms. Different fibers have distinct effects on the gut and on our overall health. For starters, some fibers are small compounds (e.g., fructans and galacto-oligosaccharides, also known as GOS, which are FODMAP fibers), and some fibers are long compounds (e.g., resistant starches, found in cooked and cooled rice and potatoes, like cold potato salad or rice salad). The size of the fiber affects how quickly and where our gut microbes will ferment the fiber and how much gas they create. Your tolerance or intolerance to different fibers depends on how your microbes interact with the fiber you eat, as well as how the type of fiber may affect your gut itself.

There are three key characteristics of fibers:

1. Solubility (ability to mix with water)
2. Degree and rate of fermentation (where and how fast microbes consume them)
3. Viscosity and gel formation (ability to thicken and become gel-like)

Insoluble fibers, which do not mix with water, are common IBS triggers. They are contained in the skins of fruits and veggies and especially in wheat bran, and they can act as an irritant in the colon, particularly for those with IBS. Wheat bran stimulates mucus production in the colon, irritating the gut lining and resulting in enhanced colonic motility, ultimately leading to diarrhea in IBS.

Soluble fibers, on the other hand—which are found in the flesh of fruits and veggies, in legumes, and in oats—help improve IBS symptoms. But it gets a bit tricky, as some small-chain soluble fibers (fructans and GOS) are also well-known IBS triggers. Fructans and GOS (aka the FODMAP fiber sources found in wheat, garlic, onion, cashews, pistachios, and legumes) are rapidly fermentable, meaning microbes enjoy them like fast foods. These FODMAP fibers can have prebiotic effects, which means they can help feed our "good" bacteria, or health-promoting gut microbes. So even though fructans and GOS are sources of FODMAPs, *they should be consumed in the diet if tolerated* due to their potential positive effects.

Let's look at two other sources of soluble fiber that tend to be well tolerated in IBS. Beta-glucan, a long-chain fiber found in oats, is also gel forming, and this property helps slow digestion in the gut, aiding with blood sugar management. Another benefit of beta-glucan is that it helps reduce blood cholesterol levels, a known risk factor for heart disease.

We often recommend taking a psyllium husk supplement as a starter intervention for IBS. Psyllium husk is a soluble fiber that has excellent evidence for its use in treating IBS symptoms. It helps improve the symptoms of both diarrhea *and* constipation. Psyllium may work well in IBS because of its capacity to hold water and resist the dehydrating effects of the large intestine. Unlike most soluble fibers, psyllium husk is associated with little to no fermentation (microbes are unable to consume it and create gas), which allows it to remain in the colon to help normalize the stool. It can soften hard stools for easier passage, and its gel-forming ability also allows it to improve loose stools and reduce urgency. Dosing starts at around 5 grams per day and can increase to 10 grams per day. See the Resources for our favorite psyllium husk options.

Most people do not eat enough fiber. The average American falls short, consuming only about 15 grams per day, compared to the recommended levels: 21–25 grams/day for adult women; 30–38 grams/day for adult men.

Because the IBS gut is highly sensitive, increase your dietary fiber intake *slowly*, starting by adding 3–5 grams per day more than is contained in your baseline diet. For example, if your baseline diet has about 10 grams of fiber daily, increase your intake to 13–15 grams of fiber per day during the initial week. If this increase is well tolerated, then add another 3–5 grams of fiber per day the following week. Eventually, your fiber intake should be close to the recommended level.

Many fiber-rich foods are also lower in common triggers (such as FODMAPs). These may be better tolerated initially. See Table 10 for IBS-friendly fiber-rich foods to try first.

TABLE 10. IBS-FRIENDLY FIBER-RICH FOODS

Gentle fiber food	Serving size	Amount of fiber (grams)
Kiwifruit, green	2 medium	4 g
Cooked oatmeal	1 cup cooked	4 g
Russet potato w/skin	1 large	5 g
Raspberries	1/4 cup	2 g
Canned pumpkin	1/3 cup	2.5 g
Canned chickpeas	1/4 cup	4 g
Chia seeds	1 tablespoon	5 g
Carrots	1 cup, chopped	4 g
Orange	1 medium	3 g

Source: USDA FoodData Central and food labels

The bottom line: Fiber inherently is good for us and our gut microbes, and most of us don't eat enough of it. But fiber tolerance varies in IBS—what works for someone else may not work for you. If your diet falls short on this important nutrient, start adding the IBS-friendly fiber-rich foods outlined in Table 10.

7. *Try Cutting Out Spicy Foods*

Several studies have shown that spicy food is associated with IBS symptoms in some people, and more frequently in women with IBS. Capsaicin, found in hot peppers, may be the primary culprit. The science is a bit mixed in this area. It appears that while capsaicin can increase GI transit and contribute to IBS-associated pain, this occurs in individuals who don't eat it often. Those who more regularly consume capsaicin in foods appear to experience *reduced* abdominal pain after consuming it. It's possible that regularly eating spicy foods actually desensitizes receptors in the gut associated with IBS pain.

The bottom line: Listen to your body, and adjust spice intake to your personal tolerance.

GUT GAME CHANGER: WHAT ABOUT GETTING TESTED FOR FOOD INTOLERANCES?

Maybe you've heard about at-home food sensitivity testing. Is it worth trying?

When it comes to food-related reactions, it is important to know the difference between food allergies and food intolerances, as discussed in Chapter 1. Unfortunately, the IgG tests that some providers or commercial companies sell on the internet have not proven very sensitive or specific in detecting a true food intolerance. Both food allergy and food intolerance tests are troubled with a high rate of false positives, which can cause people to over-restrict their diets, increase food fear and anxiety, and cause a nocebo effect (when you think the food *may* cause you harm, and therefore you have a negative response to it). This is why some allergy departments do not run wide panels of food allergy testing on people who don't present with specific allergy symptoms.

Currently, the IgG tests on the market and publicized on social media by celebrities have not been shown to reliably identify either food allergies or sensitivities. Most people produce IgG antibodies after eating food. These antibodies are not specific to a person's sensitivity, although past or frequent exposure to a food may cause their levels to be higher. All this being said, interesting research is looking at the potential for a very specific food panel to test for IgG-related food intolerance in IBS. Our hope is that food intolerance testing will become easier in the near future.

Here's one of the most effective ways to test for a food intolerance: (1) limit or avoid the food (e.g., wheat) or food trigger (e.g., gluten, FODMAPs) in question for two to six weeks, (2) assess how your symptoms respond, and then (3) do a challenge or reintroduction of the food (or food trigger) to see how you feel (do this last step one food or food trigger—e.g., gluten or a specific FODMAP—at a time).

THE GENTLE DIET CLEANUP IN ACTION

Perhaps you are ready to try the gentle diet cleanup, and you wonder what this dietary and lifestyle approach might look like in the real world. First check out the additional lifestyle recommendations listed just below. Then use the one-day menu plan following that to guide you. Use the Mind Your Gut Food and Lifestyle Tracker in the Resources (page 318) to help you keep track of what you eat and drink and any symptoms you may observe.

Additional Lifestyle Recommendations

- Move your body! Engage in regular exercise as your body allows and enjoys—such as yoga, walking, swimming, biking.
- Make relaxation and stress management a priority (see Chapters 2, 3, and 4 for tips).
- Create positive sleep habits by aiming for seven to nine hours of shut-eye per night. Your body (including the gut microbes within) benefits from adequate sleep time for mental and physical health.

Gentle Diet Cleanup Sample Menu Plan

Breakfast

Oatmeal topped with strawberries, walnuts, and a
spoonful of ground flaxseed

Coffee or tea per tolerance

Low-fat yogurt (use lactose-free if lactose intolerant)

½ English muffin with peanut butter

Glass of water

Lunch

Baked chicken with roasted (peeled) potatoes, green
beans, and carrots (season with salt, pepper, and
extra-virgin olive oil)

Grapes and a piece of dark chocolate

Glass of water

Dinner

Roasted salmon, white rice, roasted eggplant, and
tomatoes drizzled with extra-virgin olive oil

Multigrain dinner roll

Glass of water

Snack

Cheddar cheese

Handful of oat-based crackers

Glass of water

Snack

Banana Pumpkin Blender Muffin (see recipe, page 289)

Glass of water

If you decide to try this gentle approach, give it a good go for about four weeks. If you don't find that it helps adequately with your IBS symptoms, you can move on to limiting FODMAP carbohydrates, which can be very effective. As a reminder, always discuss dietary changes with your health-care team first.

THE LOW-FODMAP DIET: AN INTRODUCTION

If you've read anything about IBS and diet, you've likely encountered the term "FODMAPs." (And if you've ever had gas after eating beans, congratulations, you've experienced FODMAPs firsthand!) As a reminder, "FODMAP" is an abbreviation for "fermentable oligosaccharides, disaccharides, monosaccharides, and polyols." That's a mouthful to describe a certain group of small sugars and fibers that are commonly poorly absorbed by the gut, and that trigger GI distress in IBS. In fact, a low-FODMAP diet has been shown to offer IBS symptom resolution in up to 80 percent of patients. This nutritional approach is far more effective than most IBS medications.

FODMAPs have two key effects in the gut. One, they pull water into the gut, stretching it. Two, they become fast food for the gut microbes that live in the colon. When microbes feast on FODMAP carbohydrates, they produce gas—often lots of gas—along with other compounds and acid. The aftermath of FODMAPs in an IBS gut is often cramping, pain, diarrhea, and, in some, constipation. Not fun!

In clinical practice, there are two approaches to applying a low-FODMAP diet: a full three-phase elimination diet or a less complicated, FODMAP-flexible approach. The decision about which path to try first can be guided by your health-care team. Generally, the three-phase elimination approach is for those with more severe and debilitating IBS symptoms and who have not struggled with disordered eating. A FODMAP-flexible approach might be better for someone with less control over what food choices are available to them (like a college student), or for someone with other food intolerances or allergies, as it is less restrictive. The final two sections of this chapter describe each of these methods in turn.

GUT GAME CHANGER: BE FLEXIBLE

If food fear or disordered eating is a concern for you and your health-care team, don't worry. The brain-gut behavioral therapies outlined in Chapters 2, 3, and 4 offer many options for symptom improvement for those who are not best suited to try nutritional strategies. Having flexibility with yourself and your treatment plan is key!

THE LOW-FODMAP ELIMINATION DIET: THREE PHRASES

The low-FODMAP elimination diet involves a three-phase approach: the elimination phase, the reintroduction phase, and the personalization phase. Here's the breakdown.

Phase 1: Elimination

In phase 1, all high-FODMAP foods are removed from the diet in an effort to calm digestive symptoms. The goal is to find suitable low-FODMAP substitutions that you will enjoy and that will nourish you. See Table 11 for a list of high-FODMAP foods to eliminate, and for the many low-FODMAP foods that will play a starring role in your menus instead. This phase is best applied with the guidance of a registered dietitian who has a solid knowledge base of the low-FODMAP diet, but we will outline the key facets of the diet to get you started.

Mind Your Gut

TABLE 11. HIGH- AND LOW-FODMAP-
CONTAINING FOODS

Food group	High FODMAP (eliminate)	Low FODMAP (eat)
Fruits	Apple, apricot, avocado (>4 slices), banana (ripe > a few slices), blackberries, cherries, currants, dates, figs, grapes, mango, nectarine, peach, pear, persimmon, plums, prunes, watermelon	Avocado (3 slices), banana (just green or unripe: medium-sized; ripe: a few slices), banana chips, blueberries, cantaloupe, clementine, coconut (fresh and dried), cranberries (raw), dragon fruit, guava, honeydew (small wedge), kiwifruit (gold and green), lemon, lime, orange, papaya, passionfruit, pineapple, plantain, pomegranate arils (handful), raisins or dried cranberries (limit to 1 tablespoon), raspberries, rhubarb, starfruit, strawberries (handful)
Vegetables	Artichoke, asparagus, beets (fresh), bell pepper (red, orange, yellow: >4–5 slices), Brussels sprouts, cauliflower, celery, fennel bulb, garlic, leek bulb, most mushrooms, onion, peas, sauerkraut, savoy cabbage, scallion (bulb or white part), shallots, snow peas, squash (acorn, butternut, delicata), sugar snap peas, sweet potato (> a half, small)	Arugula, bamboo shoots, bean sprouts, beets (canned or pickled), bell pepper (green), bell pepper (red, orange, yellow: <4–5 slices), bok choy, broccoli (florets), cabbage (common and red), capers, carrots, cassava, celeriac, chili pepper, collard greens, corn (½ cob or canned), cucumber, edamame, eggplant, endive, ginger,

Vegetables continued		green beans, jicama, kale, leek (green part only), lettuce, olives, oyster mushrooms, parsnip, potatoes (white and red skin), pumpkin (canned), radish, rutabaga, scallion (green part only), seaweed, spinach, squash (spaghetti, pattypan, kabocha), sweet potato (half, small), Swiss chard, taro root, tomatillos, tomatoes (canned or a few slices fresh), turnip, water chestnuts, watercress, zucchini (5–6 slices)
Proteins	Most legumes (black beans, kidney beans, soybeans, white beans) Hummus, falafel, most veggie burgers, silken tofu, soy milk made with whole soybean Some nuts such as pistachios, cashews, or larger servings in general Protein foods marinated with onion or garlic flesh (e.g., marinated fish, chicken, tofu)	Beef, chicken, edamame, eggs, firm tofu, fish, lamb, pork, tempeh, turkey, shellfish Canned chickpeas up to ¼ cup Canned or boiled lentils up to ⅓ cup Nuts (limit to one handful): almonds, Brazil nuts, chestnuts, hazelnuts, peanuts, pecans, pine nuts, walnuts Almond butter (1 tablespoon), peanut butter (2 tablespoons) Seeds (limit to one handful): chia, flax, hemp, poppy, pumpkin, sesame, sunflower

Grains and starches	Most wheat-based products: rolls, bread, pasta, flour tortillas Wheat-based grains: einkorn, emmer, farro, kamut, spelt Barley, rye Soy flour Pumpernickel bread	Corn tortillas Slow-leavened sourdough wheat or slow-leavened sourdough spelt bread Buckwheat Corn and potato starch Millet Oatmeal, oat bran Pasta: rice, corn, quinoa blends Polenta Quinoa (black, red, white) Rice (whole-grain and flour) Soba noodles Sorghum Teff flour
Fats	Those with added garlic and onion flesh or other FODMAP ingredients	Most oils and butter
Dairy and dairy substitutes	Buttermilk, cow's milk, goat's milk Ice cream Yogurt Cottage cheese, ricotta cheese Soy milk (made with whole soybean), oat milk	Lactose-free varieties of milk, cottage cheese, ice cream, and yogurt Butter Hard and aged cheeses: cheddar, havarti, Swiss, Parmesan Some soft cheeses: mozzarella, feta, goat (chevre), queso fresco

Dairy and dairy substitutes continued		Coconut-based cheese and coconut-based yogurt Plant-based milks: almond, coconut, hemp, rice, macadamia, quinoa
Other	Additives: agave, chicory root extract, inulin Rum Kombucha Fennel or chamomile tea	Sweeteners: maple syrup, gluten-free flour blends for cooking (avoid those with soy and bean flour options) Corn and potato starch Nutritional yeast Tea: peppermint, green, white, or black Wine: dry white or red Vodka, tequila, whiskey

You may have noticed that slow-leavened sourdough wheat or spelt bread is low-FODMAP. When bread is made using a slow fermentation process and a live sourdough culture, the live yeast and bacteria in the culture consume some of the wheat-based fructans, resulting in a lower-FODMAP-containing bread. The microbes also ferment some of the wheat-based gluten but not enough for the bread to be considered gluten-free.

To apply a low-FODMAP elimination diet as seamlessly as possible, Chapter 6 covers:

- Label reading (to help identify FODMAPs on a food label and logos that certify a product is low-FODMAP)
- Menu-planning tips (to provide personal meal ideas, including many of your favorite foods and their substitutes)

- Grocery shopping tips (to help you find brand-name low-FODMAP foods in the market or online)

....

DIGESTIBLE DETAIL: SIZE MATTERS

Food intolerance reactions are driven by the amount consumed. Larger amounts of FODMAPs will likely result in more digestive symptoms while small amounts less so. For instance, a splash of cow's milk in coffee provides a very small amount of lactose. Even for those with a history of lactose intolerance, a splash of milk is often well tolerated, even on a low-FODMAP elimination diet. Similarly, small portions of wheat, such as the amount contained in a handful of crackers, is low enough in FODMAPs to be considered low-FODMAP.

....

We also provide food brand suggestions in the Resources section. Research to test foods for FODMAP content is ongoing, and digital apps to provide updated FODMAP food lists are being developed. Our favorite app is from Monash FODMAP. It is widely available in app stores; we have it listed along with other apps for IBS in the Resources section.

Watch Out for Hidden FODMAPs

Since you're making valiant efforts to go low-FODMAP, make sure you're not thwarted by hidden FODMAPs. These are often found in snacks and prepared food products. If they remain in your diet, they will prevent you from getting the most symptom benefit from phase 1. Sometimes FODMAPs lurk in food products that you may have inadvertently missed when you purchased them. Common culprits include granola or snack bars (which can contain FODMAPs in the form of chicory root, inulin, dates, or honey), smoothies (chicory root, cashew milk, soy milk, agave syrup), kefir and yogurt (chicory root, inulin), salad dressing (onion, garlic), broth (onion, garlic), seasoned snacks (legume flours, garlic, onion), and some probiotic supplements, which often contain FODMAP prebiotic sources (chicory root, inulin, fructo-oligosaccharides).

How Long Do I Stay in the Elimination Phase?

Phase 1 is typically applied for two to six weeks. If your symptoms are minimal after two weeks, you can move on to phase 2. Most people require about four weeks in phase 1 to get maximum symptom reduction, as it takes a week or so to fully assimilate the diet into your life.

By the end of phase 1, you may notice one of the following:

1. Your IBS symptoms are manageable, and you feel great—yay! You have learned that FODMAPs are an IBS symptom trigger for you.
2. You notice some reduction in symptoms but feel only partially better. Good: you have learned that FODMAPs may be a part of your IBS symptom picture. There's a little more work to do to figure out the rest.
3. You don't notice any change in your IBS symptoms. That's a bummer, but now you know that FODMAPs are probably not a symptom trigger, and you can move in a different direction with your treatment plan.

If you didn't notice that your digestive distress improved at all from the low-FODMAP elimination diet and you feel confident you were applying it correctly, it's time to go back to your regular diet and work with your health-care team to find another treatment approach. The good news here is that research has shown that many other treatments can help your IBS. In fact, one study comparing the efficacy of a low-FODMAP diet to using gut-directed hypnosis found that both interventions improved gut symptoms similarly. So if diet isn't your answer, we've got more science-backed solutions for you.

Phase 2: Reintroduction

Once you've been sticking to your list of FODMAP-rich foods to avoid for some time, we have great news for you! It's time for a more expansive diet. The reintroduction phase is a critical step in helping you live a full life with IBS. So let's get you eating as much variety as possible.

If your IBS symptoms improved during phase 1 of the diet, it's time to learn which FODMAPs are your triggers. Identifying your personal triggers can be quite empowering, as you will finally know what was instigating your digestive woes and what foods can be added back to your plate.

The reintroduction phase is a systematic process. (So don't load up on garlicky pasta with ice cream for dessert just yet!) FODMAPs are added very gradually back to the diet—that means one FODMAP subtype at a time, and only one food at a time. For example, for the first week or two you might only reintroduce foods containing lactose, slowly adding cow's milk for a few days before trying yogurt. After that, you might move on to foods with excess fructose, followed by the fructans, galacto-oligosaccharides, and polyols (both sorbitol and mannitol). (See page 31 in Chapter 1 for greater detail on each FODMAP subtype.) If you react to a food, remember, the goal of this important phase is not to make you feel miserable again but rather to help you identify the foods that need to take a back seat in your diet.

Steps of the Reintroduction Phase

1. Remain on your baseline low-FODMAP elimination diet.

2. Test your tolerance to only one FODMAP subtype (e.g., foods containing lactose or foods containing excess fructose, etc.) at a time. Take about one week to re-introduce each FODMAP subtype, and within that, take about three days to add back one specific FODMAP-containing food in incremental amounts.

3. Keep FODMAP reintroduction portions in line with what you would normally eat. There is no need to over-eat a FODMAP food just to see what it might do.

4. Try to incorporate the test food into your low-FODMAP diet for at least three consecutive days, increasing the portion as outlined below to confirm tolerance.

5. If you exhibit undesirable symptoms such as severe bloating, pain, diarrhea, or constipation (i.e., the return of your IBS symptoms), stop the reintroduction of that food and give your gut a rest.

6. Only resume the reintroduction of FODMAPs when your gut is settled for at least three days in a row.

Jeff is ready to start the reintroduction phase of the low-FODMAP elimination diet. He will begin by reintroducing lactose. Jeff maintains his low-FODMAP elimination diet while adding cow's milk to his diet. On the first day of his lactose reintroduction, Jeff adds ½ cup of milk to his breakfast meal. He will use the Mind Your Gut Food and Lifestyle Tracker (found in the Resources section) to track any symptoms he may experience with the milk reintroduction.

Jeff doesn't notice any GI symptoms on day one. The next day, he increases the milk portion to 1 cup at breakfast; he notices a slight uptick in gas about two hours after consuming the milk. The symptoms he experienced were not painful and did not resemble an IBS flare. Jeff remembers that adding back FODMAPs can increase intestinal gas, but as long as it's not painful or troublesome, he can move on with the reintroduction process. The next day, he drinks 12 ounces of milk at breakfast. Two hours later, Jeff notes some cramping gas and has to use the toilet urgently with diarrhea. Jeff's dietitian suggests that as he continues with the personalization phase of his diet, he limit his milk consumption to no more than 1 cup per meal. Alternatively, Jeff can try using lactase pills (digestive enzyme pills that can help aid lactose digestion) when he consumes milk or milk products to see if they offer improved tolerance with portions of milk greater than 1 cup. Because tolerance to FODMAPs can change over time, Jeff's dietitian suggests that he test his tolerance to larger portions (greater than 1 cup) of lactose again in a few months.

For the next reintroduction trial, Jeff decides to test his tolerance to mannitol. For this reintroduction (and all the remaining ones), Jeff will follow his baseline low-FODMAP elimination diet. That means he will discontinue eating any of his "passed" FODMAP-containing foods (in this case, lactose) until he starts phase 3 of the diet, the personalization phase.

Ready to get started? There is no special order in which you should reintroduce FODMAP subtypes. Two research studies that assessed likely triggers during reintroduction found that fructans, GOS, and mannitol were the most common. But given that IBS is very individual, through trial and error you will find what works and what doesn't for *you*. You may decide to start with the FODMAP subtype you most miss, or start with the one that contains foods you think you tolerate.

Suggested Foods and Portion Sizes for Reintroduction

During the reintroduction phase, it is important to select foods that contain *only* the FODMAP subtype you are testing. Some foods contain more than one subtype, such as apples, which contain sorbitol and excess fructose. Here is a list of some foods (and portions) that would be appropriate for FODMAP reintroduction. Note that, unless otherwise specified, the portion sizes are based on the food's raw form. You may cook these foods, but measure them out when the food is raw to ensure suitable portion size. All veggies and fruits listed are medium in size.

Lactose

½ cup (120 ml) cow's milk

¾ cup plain cow's milk yogurt (without high-fructose corn syrup or other FODMAP ingredients)

Excess fructose

½ mango

1 tablespoon honey

½ cup sugar snap peas

Polyols

Mannitol

½ cup button mushrooms

⅓ cup chopped cauliflower

1 cup diced sweet potato

Sorbitol

5 blackberries

½ yellow peach

½ avocado

Fructans

(we recommend doing reintroduction trials
for wheat, garlic, and onion separately to gauge
tolerance or intolerance)

1 tablespoon finely chopped onion (cooked onion might be better tolerated for the initial trial)

½ clove of garlic

1–2 slices traditional wheat bread without other FOD-MAP ingredients

Galacto-oligosaccharides

½ cup cooked beans, such as black beans, kidney beans, soybeans

---

GUT GAME CHANGER: LESS STRESS WHEN ADDING MORE

Stress-related and FODMAP-induced symptoms can mimic each other, so do the reintroduction phase of the low-FODMAP diet when your life is less busy or stressed. A more relaxed environment will provide greater insight into food triggers.

On the first day of reintroduction, start with the portion size listed above. On the second day, if you did not experience a significant uptick in symptoms, you can double the portion. And again, on day three, if you have not experienced undesirable or painful symptoms, triple the portion size from that listed above.

It's not necessary to reintroduce a portion size that exceeds what you normally would consume, so if the second day's portion is what you'd typically eat, maintain that amount for day three.

Sample Three-Day Reintroduction Trials

Let's see what three-day reintroduction trials might look like using the various FODMAP subtypes (Tables 12–19). These sample trials list specific foods, but if you really dislike, say, cauliflower and wouldn't eat it under normal circumstances, you can of course substitute one of the other mannitol foods listed above.

TABLE 12. LACTOSE REINTRODUCTION
(COW'S MILK)

DAY 1	DAY 2	DAY 3
Add 1/2 cup cow's milk to your baseline low-FODMAP diet	If there is no significant reaction to the initial lactose reintroduction, add 1 cup cow's milk to your baseline low-FODMAP diet	If there is no significant reaction to the second lactose reintroduction, add 1 1/2 cups cow's milk to your baseline low-FODMAP diet.

TABLE 13. MANNITOL REINTRODUCTION
(CAULIFLOWER)

DAY 1	DAY 2	DAY 3
Add 1/3 cup cauliflower to your baseline low-FODMAP diet	If there is no significant reaction to the initial mannitol reintroduction, add 2/3 cup cauliflower to your baseline low-FODMAP diet	If there is no significant reaction to the second mannitol reintroduction, add 1 cup cauliflower to your baseline low-FODMAP diet

TABLE 14. SORBITOL REINTRODUCTION
(BLACKBERRIES)

DAY 1	DAY 2	DAY 3
Add 5 blackberries to your baseline low-FODMAP diet	If there is no significant reaction to the initial sorbitol reintroduction, add 10 blackberries to your baseline low-FODMAP diet	If there is no significant reaction to the second sorbitol reintroduction, add 15 blackberries to your baseline low-FODMAP diet

TABLE 15. FRUCTAN REINTRODUCTION
(WHEAT)

As mentioned previously, to reintroduce fructans, given their variety, we encourage you to conduct *separate* trials for each of the three main fructan foods (wheat, onion, and garlic) to assess tolerance or intolerance.

DAY 1	DAY 2	DAY 3
Add 1 slice of wheat bread to your baseline low-FODMAP diet	If there is no significant reaction to the initial wheat reintroduction, add 2 slices of wheat bread to your baseline low-FODMAP diet	If there is no significant reaction to the second wheat reintroduction, add 3 slices of wheat bread to your baseline low-FODMAP diet

TABLE 16. FRUCTAN REINTRODUCTION
(ONION)

DAY 1	DAY 2	DAY 3
Add 1 tablespoon chopped onion (cooked may be better tolerated) to your baseline low-FODMAP diet	If there is no significant reaction to the initial onion reintroduction, add 2 tablespoons chopped onion to your baseline low-FODMAP diet	If there is no significant reaction to the second onion reintroduction, add 3 tablespoons chopped onion to your baseline low-FODMAP diet

TABLE 17. FRUCTAN REINTRODUCTION
(GARLIC)

DAY 1	DAY 2	DAY 3
Add 1/2 clove of garlic to your baseline low-FODMAP diet	If there is no significant reaction to the initial garlic reintroduction, add 1 clove of garlic to your baseline low-FODMAP diet	If there is no significant reaction to the second garlic reintroduction, add 1 1/2 cloves of garlic to your baseline low-FODMAP diet

TABLE 18. GOS REINTRODUCTION
(BEANS)

DAY 1	DAY 2	DAY 3
Add 1/2 cup cooked beans to your baseline low-FODMAP diet	If there is no significant reaction to the GOS reintroduction, add 1 cup cooked beans to your baseline low-FODMAP diet	If there is no significant reaction to the second GOS reintroduction, add 1 1/2 cups cooked beans to your baseline low-FODMAP diet

TABLE 19. EXCESS FRUCTOSE REINTRODUCTION
(HONEY)

DAY 1	DAY 2	DAY 3
Add 1 tablespoon honey to your baseline low-FODMAP diet	If there is no significant reaction to the excess fructose reintroduction, add 2 tablespoons honey to your baseline low-FODMAP diet	If there is no significant reaction to the second excess fructose reintroduction, add 3 tablespoons honey to your baseline low-FODMAP diet

During the reintroduction phase, don't forget to keep track of what you're eating and how you're feeling. This is a good time to use the Mind Your Gut Food and Lifestyle Tracker (found in the Resources) to help you identify any changes in your digestive symptoms related to adding back each food to your diet. For ease of use, copy the form in a larger version to provide adequate room for your notes.

What Is a Failed FODMAP Reintroduction?

In a failed FODMAP reintroduction, your digestive symptoms resemble an IBS flare. You will experience pain and a return of your IBS symptoms. Slight bloating and an uptick in intestinal gas do not qualify as a failed reintroduction! It is very normal to experience more gas and even a little bloating when adding FODMAPs back to your diet.

BRAIN BITE: POSTMEAL BREATHING SESSION

To help alleviate any GI sensations that may be slightly amped up as you adjust and expand your diet, try using diaphragmatic breathing for about five minutes after eating as outlined for you on page 57.

Putting into Practice What You Learned in Phase 2

Now that you understand which FODMAP types trigger your gut symptoms, you can apply the following guidelines:

If you learned that **lactose** is a trigger for you, continue to consume lactose-free milk, hard cheeses, and lactose-free yogurt, as well as low-FODMAP plant-based milks such as almond milk, hemp milk, and rice milk. Canned coconut milk (in small amounts and without added FODMAP ingredients) is another suitable dairy-free (and lactose-free) alternative.

You may try a lactase enzyme supplement to help your body digest lactose should you consume foods with lactose; see the Resources for brand names.

If you learned that **excess fructose** is a trigger, limit foods or beverages that contain ingredients with more fructose than glucose, such as apples, cherries, figs, pears, mangos, watermelon, honey, agave syrup, high-fructose corn syrup, asparagus, sugar snap peas, and rum. Consume these based on your personal tolerance.

If you learned that **sorbitol**-rich foods are a trigger, limit or avoid sugar-free gum and mints made with sorbitol. Also limit the following fruits based on your personal tolerance: apples, apricots, blackberries, cherries, nectarines, peaches, pears, and plums.

If you learned that **mannitol**-rich foods are a trigger, limit most mushrooms, cauliflower, snow peas, watermelon, and sugar-free mints or gum made with mannitol. Consume these based on your personal tolerance.

If you learned that **onion** is a trigger, limit onion. Instead, add onion flavor to your foods with shallot-infused oil, chives, the green part of scallions, and the green part of leeks.

If you learned that **garlic** is a trigger, limit garlic, and instead add garlic flavor to foods via garlic-infused oils.

If you learned that **wheat**-rich foods are a trigger, limit or avoid wheat-based foods (bread, pasta). Enjoy other wheat-free grains such as rice, oats, quinoa, and corn (polenta). Use slow-leavened sourdough wheat or spelt bread if you can tolerate it.

Like onion, wheat, and garlic, other **fructan**-rich foods may trigger your symptoms, including Brussels sprouts, dried fruits, and most beans (cannellini, kidney, pinto). Limit these per your personal tolerance.

If you learn that **GOS**-rich foods are a trigger, minimize your bean intake to your personal tolerance. Canned lentils and canned chickpeas have lower amounts of GOS compared with other legumes. Spreading out small amounts of legumes throughout the day may be better tolerated than consuming a large portion at one time. If you want to keep eating beans, you can try taking the supplement alpha-galactosidase, which has been shown to enhance tolerance to beans or other GOS-containing foods in some individuals with IBS. See the Resources for brands.

BRAIN BITE: REINTRODUCTION ANXIETY

It is not uncommon for the reintroduction phase to provoke a bit of anxiety. We get it! If you are finally feeling better, why rock the boat? Well . . . as you have read, the desire to avoid the science-based benefits of reintroduction are likely driven by anxiety. Take a few minutes to revisit some of the anxiety-management and relaxation strategies that you have found helpful. Prior to a meal, engage in one of the Five Strategies for Calm introduced in Chapter 2. Then hop back into the kitchen to reacquaint yourself with FODMAP-containing foods.

Phase 3: Personalization

After you have identified which FODMAP foods are triggers and which ones you can tolerate, move into the personalization phase. This is when you reinstate FODMAPs that you can tolerate and develop your own individualized, moderate-FODMAP diet. As you experiment with adding foods back to your diet, you will learn more about what works for your body and what doesn't. Remember, FODMAP-containing foods are not "bad for you," but some FODMAP-containing foods in large amounts may trigger GI woes. If you find that your IBS flares as you add foods, simply undergo the elimination phase for a day or two to calm the gut, and try again to reintroduce foods to assess your tolerance. Sometimes it's not the specific FODMAP-containing food on its own that triggers symptoms but rather eating a large portion or combining it with other FODMAP foods.

THE FODMAP-FLEXIBLE APPROACH

As discussed earlier in the chapter, the FODMAP-flexible approach is a less detailed and less restrictive way to modify FODMAPs in your diet. Although this approach has not yet been formally evaluated in a research setting, many dietitians use it in clinical practice with great results for people living with IBS. Unlike the more formal low-FODMAP elimination diet—which in general is implemented the same way for each person—FODMAP-flexible relies more on the individual's typical diet and symptom history to ascertain which foods are the most likely triggers. The dietitian will use this information to guide what foods to modify or eliminate.

In the FODMAP-flexible approach, typically just a few items that are very rich in FODMAPs are eliminated or reduced. After following this adjustment for a week or two, you and your health provider can evaluate the effectiveness of the change and adjust as needed. It's generally a quick process to assess for FODMAP sensitivity. This, as we call it in the science community, is a "bottom-up" approach, one that limits just a few specific foods while monitoring symptom response, and it works well for many folks.

Let's look at three examples of how someone might adjust their routine with a FODMAP-flexible approach. Often just one or two changes go a long way.

1. Susie eats a well-balanced diet overall. Every day she started her morning with a large smoothie from one of her favorite local shops. Upon review of the ingredients, she discovered that the smoothie contained cashew milk, agave syrup, and about 4 cups of fruit (a mix

of mango, strawberries, apple, and banana). The suspect FODMAPs were in the cashew milk (fructans and GOS), agave syrup (excess fructose), mango (excess fructose), apple (excess fructose and sorbitol), and perhaps the banana, depending on its ripeness (ripe bananas contain fructans).

Susie realized that her daily smoothie had FODMAP overload! She decided to start making her breakfast smoothie at home instead, using suitable low-FODMAP ingredients such as blueberries, pineapple, and lactose-free yogurt. This one adaptation in her diet was enough to dramatically reduce Susie's overall FODMAP load while the rest of her diet stayed the same. Susie noted significant symptom benefits and decided to continue making her own smoothies most of the time. She also became more mindful of the ingredients in the smoothies she selected when purchasing one at a shop.

Well-meaning foodies and individuals seeking gut health often create smoothies with copious amounts of fruits and vegetables. The sheer quantity—as well as the types—of fruit and veggies can put the smoothie over the top in FODMAP content. Modifying the portions of fruits or vegetables can lower FODMAP intake to a more tolerable level. (Does this description have you craving a delicious smoothie? Check out the Oatmeal Cookie Smoothie recipe on page 308!)

2. Elsie is an elderly woman who lives alone. Her IBS-D had been a challenge lately, and she was looking for some diet guidance. She was on medications for blood pressure, which she took with applesauce to help her swallow the pills. She also liked to sip on apple juice throughout the day. The apple juice and applesauce, two FODMAP-rich foods, were taking center stage in Elsie's diet. Apples are rich in sorbitol and excess fructose, both of which can contribute to diarrhea. Elsie was encouraged to switch to lactose-free yogurt to accompany her medications, and to try cranberry juice made with low-FODMAP ingredients instead of apple juice. The rest of her diet remained the same. This simple

adjustment provided significant relief. She experienced much less diarrhea, and she was thrilled.

3. Jamison is a barista with IBS who noticed an uptick in his gas and bloating. As part of his work benefits, specialty coffees were free. Jamison had been enjoying two large soy lattes per day. Most soy milk is made from whole soybeans, making it a high-FODMAP option.

Jamison was advised to substitute almond milk (a low-FODMAP milk) for the soy milk to reduce his FODMAP load. This slight adjustment was enough for Jamison to feel his gut settle without affecting his enjoyment of his favorite beverage.

DIGESTIBLE DETAIL: THE IMPORTANCE OF ASKING ABOUT INGREDIENTS

Keep in mind that FODMAPs often hide in prepared foods and beverages. When dining out from home, we usually select foods based on the menu description, which often doesn't display all the ingredients. It's okay to ask specific questions about the peanut butter (it might contain honey), or the marinade (hidden onion/garlic), or sweeteners (agave syrup) that may contain one of your key FODMAP triggers. Your health and wellness are important, and asking for clarifications doesn't mean you're posing an inconvenience. When it comes to your stress levels around food, learning about ingredients is a controllable stressor. Knowing that the foods you choose are likely to leave your gut feeling happy and satisfied—not hungry or seeking the loo—can afford instant relief.

Table 20 provides a list of common high-FODMAP foods that may be modified in a FODMAP-flexible approach.

TABLE 20. THE HIGHEST-FODMAP FOODS

Grains	Wheat and rye
Vegetables	Cauliflower, garlic, leek, onion, most mushrooms
Dairy	Milk and traditional yogurt
Fruit	Apples, pears, dried fruits
Legumes	Beans, such as soybeans, most soy milk, kidney beans, black beans

Whether you start with the gentle diet cleanup, the low-FODMAP elimination diet, or the FODMAP-flexible approach, notice how food feels in your intestines *and* how changing your diet affects your psyche. Remember, the nutritional approach you engage in should benefit both your gut and your mind for whole-body well-being.

CHAPTER 6

IBS-FRIENDLY MENU PLANNING, GROCERY SHOPPING, AND LABEL READING

What does low-FODMAP look like out in the real world? We're glad you asked! We're going to equip you with a week's worth of menus for a low-FODMAP diet—plus vegetarian and vegan options and kid-friendly meals—so you'll never be left wondering what to plan for dinner.

One of Kate's favorite sayings is "A balanced plate makes a balanced body." When you consume a variety of plant-based foods—such as whole grains and starchy vegetables for energy, vibrant and colorful fruits and vegetables for fiber and good nutrition, healthy fats, and satiating protein—your body *and* your gut microbiota will thrive. A balanced-plate eating pattern keeps you comfortably full, helps regulate your blood sugar, and ensures you get the nutrients you need. As you start with diet modifications to potentially help minimize digestive distress, whether you follow the gentle diet cleanup or the low-FODMAP elimination diet, the balanced menus in this chapter and the gut-friendly recipes in Appendix I will fit both approaches.

LOW-FODMAP ELIMINATION DIET: SEVEN-DAY MENU PLANNER

Let's look at a week of menus to help illustrate how to plan your plate while staying on a low-FODMAP elimination diet. (Remember, the low-FODMAP diet is a three-phase approach, and the elimination phase is just the beginning, lasting two to six weeks max.)

To provide general guidance for balancing your plate, protein-rich foods are identified with (P); colorful, fiber-rich fruits or vegetables with (FR) or (V); healthy fats with (HF); and starchy vegetables and grains with (E) for energy promoting.

When planning snacks, try to include some fiber (from whole-grain crackers or tortilla chips, fruit, or veggies) and protein. These key combos of nutrients will keep you full. Feel free to season your food with a dash of salt and pepper to taste unless advised otherwise by your health-care provider.

DIGESTIBLE DETAIL: DON'T FORGET THE PROTEIN

Note that most low-FODMAP plant-based milks, such as rice milk and almond milk, do not offer up much in the way of protein. In fact, most provide only 1–2 grams of protein per cup. Compare that with lactose-free cow's milk, which provides 8 grams of protein per cup. If you use these nondairy milks, include other protein-rich sources in your meals, such as nut butter (almond or peanut butter), firm tofu, eggs, poultry, or allowed legumes.

DAY 1

Breakfast

Veggie omelet made with 2 eggs (P) and filled with baby
  spinach (V), ¼ cup chopped green bell pepper (V), and
  ¼ cup grated cheddar cheese (P)
Enjoy with hash browns (E) made or drizzled with
  extra-virgin olive oil (HF)

Lunch

Turkey avocado arugula sammie: 2 slices slow-leavened
  sourdough wheat bread (E), sliced home-cooked-style
  turkey breast (P), arugula (V), slice tomato (V), and
  2 slices avocado (FR, HF)
Enjoy with an orange (FR) and a cup of lactose-free
  vanilla yogurt (P)

Dinner

Baked salmon (P) with baked russet potato (E) drizzled
  with extra-virgin olive oil (HF) and topped with
  broccoli florets (V) and sliced carrots (V)
Enjoy with 5 strawberries (FR) and a handful of
  dark-chocolate-dipped almonds (P)

Snacks

Scoop of Low-FOD Lemony Hummus (page 303)
  (HF, P) along with a handful of whole-grain
  low-FODMAP crackers (E)
Banana Pumpkin Blender Muffin (page 289) (E, FR, V,
  HF), topped with 1 tablespoon almond butter (HF, P)

DAY 2

Breakfast

Morning Oat Bowl (page 292) (E, FR, HF)
1 cup suitable lactose-free yogurt (P)

Lunch

Fiesta salad: Place a layer of brown rice (E) or quinoa (E) in a
   bowl; top with baby spinach or kale (V), shredded carrots
   (V), and 3–4 sliced cherry tomatoes (FR), along with ¼ cup
   canned chickpeas (P) and ¼ cup canned corn, drained (E);
   add a handful of crushed tortilla chips (E), and drizzle with
   fresh lime juice and extra-virgin olive oil (HF)
Enjoy with a small wedge of cantaloupe (FR)

Dinner

Shrimp sauté: In a medium skillet over medium heat,
   pan-fry shelled and deveined shrimp (P) in toasted
   sesame oil; add 1 cup broccoli florets (V) and chopped
   bok choy (V), cooking until fork-tender; sprinkle with
   soy sauce and sesame seeds (HF)
Serve over brown rice noodles (E)

Snacks

Suitable whole-grain crackers (see Resources for brand
   suggestions) (E) and cheddar cheese (P) with carrot
   sticks (V)
Peanut Butter Dark Chocolate Chip Energy Bites (page
   306) (E, P, HF)

DAY 3

Breakfast

Peanut butter–banana toast: Spread a layer of peanut
butter (P, HF) over slow-leavened sourdough wheat
toast (E); top with thinly sliced ripe banana (FR) (limit
to about ⅓ banana), 1 tablespoon sunflower seeds
(HF), and a sprinkle of cinnamon

Lunch

Carrot Ginger Soup (page 295) (V) with suitable
whole-grain low-FODMAP crackers (E) and a few slices
of cheddar cheese (P)
Enjoy with diced pineapple (FR) and a handful of
walnuts (HF)

Dinner

Firm-tofu Asian stir-fry: Sauté diced firm tofu (P) in
sesame oil over medium heat until golden-brown;
add steamed carrots (V), broccoli florets (V), and fresh
bean sprouts (V); add a splash of soy sauce and minced
fresh ginger to taste
Serve over quinoa or brown rice (E) that has been drizzled
with extra-virgin olive oil (HF)

Snacks

Oatmeal Cookie Smoothie (page 308) (E, P)
Almond Cranberry Energy Bites (page 305) (E, HF, P)

DAY 4

Breakfast

Hard-cooked egg (P) served alongside avocado toast: Toast
1–2 slices slow-leavened sourdough wheat bread (E);
spread about 1 tablespoon mashed avocado (FR, HF) over
each slice; sprinkle with chia seeds (HF), sunflower seeds
(HF), and a drizzle of extra-virgin olive oil (HF)

Enjoy with a bowl of blueberries (FR)

Lunch

Arugula (V) salad dressed with lemon juice (FR) and extra-
virgin olive oil (HF); add some protein: ¼ cup canned
chickpeas (P), ⅓ cup canned lentils (P), or baked
chicken (P)

Low-FODMAP roll (E) (see Resources for brand suggestions)

Enjoy with ½ cup lactose-free yogurt (P), topped with a
few sliced strawberries (FR) and a sprinkle of chopped
pecans (HF)

Dinner

Italian pasta night: Boil up a serving of gluten-free pasta
(E); top with ground chicken or lean ground beef (P) that
has been simmered in low-FODMAP marinara (FR)

Enjoy with a side salad (V) composed of lettuce, tomato,
carrots, and cucumber and dressed with a low-FODMAP
dressing (HF) such as Maple Dijon Dressing (page 309)
(see Resources for brand suggestions for marinara sauce
and salad dressing)

Snacks

Handful of tortilla chips (E), carrot sticks (V), and ¼ cup
Low-FOD Lemony Hummus (page 303) (P)

Yogurt parfait: ½ cup lactose-free low-FODMAP yogurt (P),
sliced kiwifruit (FR), and ¼ cup Low-FODMAP Seedy
Granola (page 288) (E, HF)

DAY 5

Breakfast

Overnight oats: Fill a small mason jar with ½ cup rolled
oats (E), 2 teaspoons chia seeds (HF), and 1 cup milk of
choice (lactose-free cow's milk (P), rice milk, or almond milk);
add a sprinkle of cinnamon and 1 teaspoon maple syrup;
stir ingredients together well and refrigerate overnight
Top with low-FODMAP fruit of choice (FR)

Lunch

Power Sport Smoothie (page 308) (E, P, HF, FR)
Enjoy with a suitable low-FODMAP snack bar (see Resources)

Dinner

Grilled flank steak (P), baked russet potato (E) drizzled with
extra-virgin olive oil (HF), oven-roasted green beans (V)
Dark chocolate fondue: In a microwave-safe bowl, combine
2 tablespoons dark chocolate and 1 tablespoon peanut butter
(P, HF); microwave until melted, 15–30 seconds
Serve with 5 strawberries (FR) for dipping

Snacks

1 Banana Pumpkin Blender Muffin (page 289) (E, V, FR,
HF) and ½ cup lactose-free kefir
2 tablespoons Low-FOD Lemony Hummus (page 303) (P),
a handful of carrot sticks (V), and suitable whole-grain
crackers (see Resources)

DAY 6

Breakfast

From-the-Garden Egg Cups (page 291) (P, V)
Enjoy with a side of hash browns (E) made with
    extra-virgin olive oil (HF), and a small bowl of diced
    pineapple (FR)

Lunch

Zesty Lentil Soup (page 294) (P, HF, V, FR)
Enjoy with a handful of whole-grain, low-FODMAP
    crackers (E) and a small bowl of diced cantaloupe or an
    orange (FR)

Dinner

Pizza for one: Brush garlic-infused oil on a suitable
    low-FODMAP pizza crust (E) (see Resources); top with
    a few thin slices of tomato (FR) and ⅓ cup shredded
    mozzarella cheese (P); bake pizza as directed on package;
    remove from oven when cheese is melted and crust is
    browned, and top with fresh basil leaves (V)
Enjoy with a side salad (V) made with low-FODMAP
    veggies and topped with a low-FODMAP salad dressing;
    see recipes and Resources for inspiration on salad dressings

Snacks

Popcorn (E) and a small bowl of chopped cantaloupe or
    blueberries (FR)
Tortilla chips (E) topped with a sprinkle of shredded
    cheddar cheese (P) and served with low-FODMAP salsa
    (FR) (see Resources for brand suggestions)

DAY 7

Breakfast

Vanilla-cinnamon French toast: Whisk together 1 egg (P) and ¼ cup lactose-free milk (P); add a dash of vanilla extract and a sprinkle of cinnamon; dip 2 slices of low-FODMAP bread (E) into the mixture, and brown the bread in a nonstick skillet; top with a spoonful of suitable vanilla yogurt (P), ¼ cup low-FODMAP fruit (FR) of choice, a spoonful of chopped walnuts (HF), and a drizzle of maple syrup

Lunch

Tuna salad bowl: In a serving bowl, toss together chopped lettuce (V), carrot (V), and cucumber (V) slices; in a separate bowl, stir together canned tuna (P), a squeeze of fresh lemon juice, and 1–2 teaspoons mayonnaise; spoon on top of the veggies

Serve with a low-FODMAP roll (E) (see Resources for ideas) and an orange (FR)

Dinner

Grilled fish (P), Confetti Rice (page 301) (V, E, HF), and sautéed green beans (V)

Enjoy with a piece of dark chocolate and a handful of strawberries (FR)

Snacks

1–2 Energy Bites (either Almond Cranberry, page 305, or Peanut Butter Dark Chocolate Chip, page 306) (E, HF) and lactose-free yogurt (P)

Rice cake (E) topped with peanut butter (HF, P), a smear of strawberry jam (made *without* high-fructose corn syrup), and a sprinkle of chia seeds (HF)

DIGESTIBLE DETAIL: ADD FLAVOR WITH GARLIC- OR SHALLOT-INFUSED OIL

We love infused oils because they provide delicious garlic and onion flavor without the FODMAPs. Both garlic and onions (including shallots and leek bulbs) contain FODMAP carbohydrates called fructans. Fructans are water-soluble fibers, so when foods containing them are added to water-based liquids such as broth or tomato sauce, the fructans can release into the sauce. But this doesn't happen with oil because water and oil don't mix. When you cook with infused oil, you can get the flavors you may have been missing without fructans sneaking in. You can buy premade shallot- and garlic-infused oil to keep on hand (see Resources), or simply make some as you cook. Pour about ¼ cup extra-virgin olive oil into a skillet over medium-low heat. Add a garlic clove or two (skin removed); alternatively, add a shallot (skin removed). Let simmer until fragrant, for 3–5 minutes. Remove the flesh of the garlic or shallot from the oil, and use the oil in your recipe. Leftover homemade infused oils should be refrigerated (unlike commercial brands) and used within four days for food-safety reasons.

ADJUSTING A LOW-FODMAP EATING PLAN TO SPECIAL DIET NEEDS

Any dietary modifications should be tailored to an individual's medical history, food preferences, culture, financial resources, cooking abilities, kitchen equipment, and lifestyle. In addition to the need to calm the gut, other personal needs sometimes must be considered, such as following a vegan or vegetarian diet, or meeting the increased calorie, protein, and nutrient needs of endurance athletes and growing kiddos. The next few sections address each of these special cases.

VEGAN AND VEGETARIAN LOW-FODMAP DIETS

For those who follow a vegan or vegetarian diet, adhering to a low-FODMAP plan may be a bit more challenging. This is because most (not all) plant-based proteins tend to be higher in FODMAPs, particularly fructans and GOS (found in beans). Vegans should stick with the lower-FODMAP plant-protein sources (such as firm tofu, edamame, tempeh, canned lentils, and canned chickpeas), suitable nuts, nut butters, and seeds. Spreading consumption of plant-based proteins over the course of the day rather than eating large quantities in one or two meals works best. Doing so will help you eat enough protein and will likely aid in better symptom control. Further, because low-FODMAP vegan protein sources are limited, we recommend following the elimination diet for no longer than two weeks.

Because most legumes are relatively high in FODMAPs, we have provided a list of lower-FODMAP plant-based protein alternatives that can make up the foundation of your protein needs while on the elimination diet. See Table 21 for low-FODMAP plant-based proteins and more.

DIGESTIBLE DETAIL: HOORAY FOR HEMP SEEDS!

Did you know that hemp seeds are a great plant-based protein? Each serving of 2 tablespoons contains 7 grams of protein! Get a protein (and flavor) boost by sprinkling hemp seeds over salads or your morning oats, or by adding them to an Energy Bite (see recipes, pages 305 and 306) or to your favorite smoothie recipe.

Mind Your Gut

TABLE 21. LOW- VERSUS HIGH-FODMAP
PLANT-BASED PROTEINS AND MORE

Low-FODMAP plant-based protein and more	High-FODMAP plant-based protein and more
Milks: Almond, hemp, macadamia, quinoa, and rice For use in recipes or in small portions, canned coconut milk (a few tablespoons) Coconut yogurt, coconut cheese	Milks: Oat and soy (made with whole soybeans)
Nuts: Almonds, chestnuts, macadamias, peanuts, pecans, pine nuts, walnuts, peanut or almond butter (limit to 1 tablespoon) Seeds: Chia, flax, hemp, poppy, pumpkin, sunflower	Nuts: Cashews, pistachios
Soy-based: Tempeh, firm tofu, edamame, soy cheese	Soy-based: Silken tofu, most soy milks
Quorn crumbles (plain)	Soy-based crumbles such as textured vegetable protein
Legumes: Canned chickpeas, canned lentils	Legumes: Kidney beans, navy beans, dried legumes

In general, if you follow a vegan or vegetarian diet, you may need to pay extra attention to ensure you obtain all the nutrition you need for health. In addition to protein, other nutrients may be reduced in a low-FODMAP vegan/vegetarian diet, including iron, vitamin B12, calcium, vitamin D, zinc, iodine, and omega-3 fats. These nutrients are outlined in Table 22, which also lists foods to help guide you in menu planning to ensure an adequate diet.

TABLE 22. NUTRIENT CONSIDERATIONS
FOR A VEGAN OR VEGETARIAN DIET

Nutrient	What it does	Where to get it (lower-FODMAP options)
Iron	Iron's main function is to bind and transport oxygen throughout the body. Plant sources contain nonheme iron, which is less well absorbed than the heme iron found in animal sources. Consuming foods rich in vitamin C (oranges, tomatoes, bell peppers) will help with the absorption of nonheme iron.	Kale Firm tofu Lentils, canned Chickpeas, canned Edamame White potatoes Sesame seeds Flaxseeds Oats
Vitamin B12	Vitamin B12 is essential for forming red blood cells and maintaining proper nervous system function. It is synthesized by microorganisms and therefore is not contained in any plant-based foods.	Vegans must supplement (recommended amount is 250 micrograms (µg)/day). Vegetarians can obtain B12 from eggs, aged cheeses, lactose-free cow's milk, and yogurt.
Calcium	Calcium is needed for the health of bones and teeth, and for normal nerve and muscle functioning.	Almonds Bok choy Broccoli florets Chia seeds Chickpeas, canned Collard greens Fortified plant-based milks: Rice, almond, or other tolerable option Firm tofu prepared with calcium Kale Tahini

Vitamin D	Vitamin D is important for the immune system, bone health, muscle function, and calcium absorption.	Sun exposure helps the body produce vitamin D, but this depends on the season, time of day, length of day, skin color, and sunscreen use.
		Mushrooms exposed to light can be a source of vitamin D (though they can be high in FODMAPs).
		For vegetarians: Fortified lactose-free milk, egg yolks
		For vegans: Fortified plant-based milks and plant-based yogurt (as tolerated)
		Consider sun exposure twice a week (10–30 minutes) and/or a vitamin D supplement.
		Note: Vitamin D2 is acceptable to vegans; vitamin D3 supplements are typically sourced from fish oil or sheep lanolin.
Zinc	This mineral is key for wound healing, immune function, and skin health.	Brazil nuts Brown rice Chickpeas, canned Lentils, canned Oatmeal Pumpkin seeds Quinoa Tempeh
Iodine	This mineral is important for thyroid hormone production.	Iodized salt Potato with skin Seaweed, nori

| Omega-3 fats | These are important for brain health, heart health, kidney function, eye health, and skin health.

Alpha-linolenic acid (ALA) is the plant-based omega-3. | Chia seeds
Chickpeas, canned
Edamame
Flaxseeds
Lentils, canned
Pecans
Walnuts |

Read on to see sample menus for vegan and vegetarian diets. Protein-rich foods are identified with (P); colorful fiber-containing fruits or vegetables with (FR) or (V); healthy fats with (HF); and starchy vegetables and grains with (E) for energy. Feel free to season your food with a dash of salt and pepper to taste unless advised otherwise by your health-care provider.

Vegan Low-FODMAP Elimination Diet:

ONE-DAY SAMPLE MENU

Breakfast

Tofu scramble made with firm tofu (P), plus spinach (V), diced green bell pepper (V), and a drizzle of extra-virgin olive oil (HF)

Energy Bite (either option, pages 305 and 306) (E, P, HF)

Coconut yogurt with Low-FODMAP Seedy Granola (page 288) (E, HF) and an orange (FR)

Lunch

Tempeh (P) stir-fry with mung bean sprouts (V), broccoli florets (V), and carrot slices (V), served with brown rice or quinoa (E) and drizzled with extra-virgin olive oil (HF)

Almond milk (fortified with calcium and vitamin D)

Strawberries (FR) and sliced kiwifruit (FR)

Dinner

Farmers' Market Pasta (page 296) (E, FR, V, HF, P)
Handful of dark-chocolate-dipped (vegan) almonds

Snacks

Almond milk (fortified with calcium and vitamin D) and
an Energy Bite (either option, pages 305 and 306) (P,
HF, E)
Trail mix made with suitable nuts and 1 tablespoon raisins

Vegetarian Low-FODMAP Elimination Diet:

ONE-DAY SAMPLE MENU

Breakfast

Lactose-free plain Greek yogurt (P) topped with a handful
of blueberries (FR), walnuts (HF), and a tablespoon of
chia seeds (HF)
¼ cup Low-FODMAP Seedy Granola (page 288) (E, HF)

Lunch

Caprese-quinoa salad: Place a scoop of quinoa (E) on a
plate; top with tomato slices (FR), a handful of baby
spinach (V), a few slices of fresh mozzarella (P), a drizzle
of extra-virgin olive oil (HF) and balsamic vinegar, and
fresh basil leaves (V)
Side of Farmers' Market Pasta (page 296) (E, FR, V, HF, P)
Raw Brownie Round (page 307) (HF, E)
1 cup diced pineapple (FR)

Dinner

Zesty Lentil Soup (page 294) (P, HF, V, FR) sprinkled
with Parmesan cheese (P)

1–2 slices of slow-leavened sourdough wheat or spelt bread (E)

Tropical fruit salad (FR) made with shredded coconut,
diced pineapple, dragon fruit, and a spoonful of
chopped walnuts (HF)

Snacks

Rice cake (E) topped with peanut butter (P, HF) and
sliced strawberries (FR)

Banana Pumpkin Blender Muffin (page 289) (E, FR, V,
HF) and a glass of lactose-free milk (P)

LOW-FODMAP DIET FOR ATHLETES

Many athletes power up with carbs because they are a key energy
source for fueling exercise—but the added carbs can increase your
FODMAP intake! If you're an athlete with IBS, see the power-packed
menu below. It provides calories in the form of carbs and healthy fats
for energy, and protein for muscle growth and repair. Protein-rich
foods are identified with (P); colorful fiber-containing fruits or vegetables with (FR) or (V); healthy fats with (HF); and starchy vegetables and grains with (E) for energy. Feel free to season your food
with a dash of salt and pepper to taste unless advised otherwise by
your health-care provider.

ONE-DAY SAMPLE MENU

Breakfast

Hash browns bowl: Cook hash browns (E) with
extra-virgin olive oil (HF); top with scrambled eggs (P),

a handful of chopped tomatoes (FR), chopped walnuts
(HF), and shredded cheddar cheese (P)
Power Sport Smoothie (page 308) (FR, P, HR)

Lunch

Baked chicken thighs (P)
Large russet potato (E)
Broccoli florets (V) sautéed in garlic-infused extra-virgin
olive oil (HF) and topped with pine nuts (HF)

Dinner

Pasta supper: Suitable gluten-free pasta (E) topped with
low-FODMAP marinara (see Resources for brand
suggestions) that has been simmered with sliced carrots
(V) and eggplant (V) and mixed with cooked ground
chicken (P) or lean ground beef (P)
Serve with a mixed salad: Baby spinach (V) tossed with
green bell pepper (V) and a handful of cherry tomatoes
(FR); drizzle with extra-virgin olive oil (HF) and lemon
juice
Orange (FR) and a handful of walnuts (HF)

Snacks

Low-lactose plain Greek yogurt (P) topped with
Low-FODMAP Seedy Granola (page 288) (HF, E) and
blueberries (FR)
1–2 slices slow-leavened sourdough wheat bread (E)
topped with peanut butter (HF, P), sliced unripe banana
(FR), and a sprinkle of chia seeds (HF)
Enjoy with a glass of lactose-free milk (P)

DIGESTIBLE DETAIL: HYDRATION AND FUELING TIPS FOR ATHLETES DURING EXERCISE

Many products that are marketed to provide hydration or energy during athletic events contain excess fructose, a FODMAP subtype. Examples include products made with honey, agave syrup, crystalline fructose, or simply fructose on its own. We encourage glucose- or sucrose-based fueling ingredients. These low-FODMAP options may keep gut symptoms at bay for the athlete with IBS.

KID-FRIENDLY LOW-FODMAP DIET

IBS does not discriminate. Abdominal pain and IBS are common in kids too. We don't recommend a full low-FODMAP elimination diet for children while they are still developing and exploring their relationship with foods. Below you will find a kid-friendly FODMAP-reduced sample menu. Protein-rich foods are identified with (P); colorful fiber-containing fruits or vegetables with (FR) or (V); healthy fats with (HF); and starchy vegetables and grains with (E) for energy. Feel free to season your child's food with a dash of salt and pepper to taste unless advised otherwise by their health-care provider.

ONE-DAY SAMPLE MENU

Breakfast

Banana Pancakes (page 293) (E, FR) topped with a smear of
butter or peanut butter (P) and a drizzle of maple syrup
1 cup milk, lactose-free if lactose intolerant (P)

Lunch

Taco lunch: Taco shells (corn-based) (E), filled with ground meat (P) that has been seasoned with a suitable low-FODMAP taco seasoning, and topped with shredded Mexican-style cheese (P) and low-FODMAP salsa (FR) (see Resources for brand suggestions)

Enjoy with an orange (FR), handful of baby carrots (V), and a cup of lactose-free yogurt (P)

Dinner

Crispy Almond Baked Chicken Tenders (page 302) (P, HF)

Confetti Rice (page 301) (E, V, HF)

Low-FOD Lemony Hummus (page 303) (P, HF) and suitable low-FODMAP whole-grain crackers (E) (see Resources)

Green beans (V) sautéed in extra-virgin olive oil (HF)

Handful of strawberries (FR)

Snacks

Lactose-free vanilla yogurt (P) with Low-FODMAP Seedy Granola (page 288) (HF, E)

Raw Brownie Round (page 307) (E, HF)

GUT GAME CHANGER: MAKE FOOD FUN

To encourage kids to have a positive relationship with food, think of FODMAP food sources as *potential triggers* rather than as "bad" versus "good" foods. Modeling positive and exploratory (and fun) language and behaviors about food in front of kids will help them form a healthy relationship with food, which ultimately helps with a healthy lifestyle. Here are some tips:

- Involve your kids in preparing a meal. This exposes them to lots of colorful fruits, veggies, and proteins.
- Avoid using food as a bribe or a punishment.
- When discussing eating, keep the focus off weight or diets. Food fuels our body and brain.
- Don't put dessert on a pedestal. Change the idea of what is considered a dessert (e.g., yogurt with a drizzle of maple syrup and a spoonful of chocolate chips).

TRICKS AND TOOLS FOR LOW-FODMAP LABEL READING

While we love foods that do not come with an ingredient list—hello, fruits and veggies, nuts and seeds—some foods that you shop for will require reading the label to be sure there are no hidden FODMAP ingredients.

Reading food packages to identify FODMAP-containing ingredients can be a little complicated. Here are a few tips to make the process easier. Ingredients on food labels are listed in order of predominance by weight. The first ingredient listed, therefore, is highest in quantity, and the last ingredient listed is lowest in quantity. In Table 23 you will find a list of common low-FODMAP ingredients, and in Table 24 you will find a list of common high-FODMAP ingredients. On the low-FODMAP elimination diet, avoid high-FODMAP ingredients. As you transition to the reintroduction and personalization phase, you will start to incorporate some high-FODMAP ingredients. As IBS reactions to food are based on the portion consumed, high-FODMAP ingredients that appear later in the ingredient list may be better tolerated as they represent only a small amount in the final food product. Consuming a lot of FODMAPs at one meal is more likely to trigger symptoms; for that reason, we encourage you to incorporate small amounts throughout the day.

TABLE 23. LOW-FODMAP INGREDIENTS

Milks: Dairy and plant-based	Lactose-free cow's milk Plant-based milks: Almond, hemp, macadamia, quinoa, rice, small amounts (3 tablespoons) of canned coconut milk
Sweeteners and other sugar-based products	Beet sugar, berry sugar, brown sugar, cane juice crystals, cane sugar, corn syrup (*not* high-fructose corn syrup), dextrose, glucose, high-maltose corn syrup, invert sugar, malt sugar, maltose, palm sugar, raw sugar, rice malt syrup, stevia, sucrose, evaporated cane sugar, table sugar
Leavening agents	Baking soda, baking powder, baker's yeast, sourdough culture
Flours and grains	Almond meal (<1/4 cup/serving), arrowroot flour, buckwheat and buckwheat flour, cornmeal, corn flour, cornstarch, green banana flour, millet and millet flour, oat bran, oats, polenta, quinoa, quinoa flour or flakes, rice (brown, basmati, white), rice bran, rice flour, sorghum flour, tapioca starch, teff, wheat starch, yam flour
Nuts and seeds	Nuts: Macadamia, peanuts, pecans, pine nuts, tiger nuts, walnuts, small handful of hazelnuts, small handful of almonds Seeds: Chia, flax, hemp, pumpkin, poppy, sesame, sunflower Tahini paste
Fats	Cocoa butter, butter, all oils
Protein	Bacon, beef, eggs, firm tofu, fish, lamb, pork, poultry, shellfish, whey protein isolate

Flavorings, herbs, spices, and condiments	Almond extract, allspice, asafetida, basil, bay leaves, black pepper, butter, capers, cardamom, cayenne pepper, chili powder (without onion or garlic), citrus juice and zest, cloves, cumin, curry leaves, dill, fennel seeds, fish sauce, five-spice blend, horseradish, lemongrass, mayonnaise, mint, mint jelly, malt extract, miso paste, mustards (without honey, onion, or garlic), nutritional yeast, oregano, oyster sauce, parsley, paprika, rosemary, saffron, sage, salt, soy sauce, star anise, tamari, tarragon, thyme, turmeric, vanilla beans or extract, vinegar, Worcestershire sauce
Thickeners	Agar agar, cornstarch, guar gum, maltodextrin, modified food starch, pectin, potato starch, soy lecithin, tapioca starch, xanthan gum
Chocolate	Cocoa, semisweet, dark

DIGESTIBLE DETAIL: GUM INGREDIENTS AND THE GUT

A quick note about gums (xanthan gum, guar gum) and pectin: You'll want to watch out for these in product ingredient lists, even though they are not technically FODMAP sources. (They are made up of long chains of carbohydrates while FODMAPs are made up of small chains.) That being said, gums and pectin are still highly fermentable in the gut and can trigger digestive distress, particularly when consumed in large amounts. They are found in many gluten-free products and plant-based milks. If your favorite products are made with gums, there is no need to completely avoid them, but if you note that they trigger symptoms, reducing the portion or limiting how often you eat them throughout the day may offer some benefits.

TABLE 24. HIGH-FODMAP INGREDIENTS

Milks: Dairy and plant-based	Cow's milk, goat's milk, sheep's milk, whey protein concentrate (may contain lactose), soy milk (made with whole soybeans), oat milk
Sweeteners	Agave syrup, crystalline fructose, fruit juice concentrate, fructose, fructose solids, high-fructose corn syrup, honey, isomalt, lactitol, maltitol, mannitol, molasses, polydextrose, sorbitol, xylitol
Flours and grains	Almond meal (>1/4 cup/serving), amaranth flour, barley and barley flour, bean flours, bulgur wheat, einkorn flour, emmer flour, freekeh, kamut, lupin flour, rye flour, soybean flour, spelt flour, wheat berries, wheat flour (all-purpose, pastry flour, white flour, whole wheat flour)
Fiber additives	Chicory root extract, inulin, fructo-oligosaccharides
Flavoring agents	Garlic, onion, "natural flavors" in products regulated by the USDA such as chicken or beef broth

USDA: United States Department of Agriculture

It's always a good idea to scan the ingredients on all product labels, even those you have read in the past, as manufacturers can change ingredients at any time. Check out Figure 6 to spot the underlined FODMAP ingredients on a food label.

To help make label reading easier and more streamlined, we have provided a sample low-FODMAP, gut-friendly grocery list in Table 25, and a detailed low-FODMAP list of brand names in the Resources section. These tools will help simplify your shopping for IBS and gut health. Note: The grocery list does not provide low-FODMAP portion sizes but rather what foods you might add to your shopping cart.

Granola Bar

Ingredients: <u>Chicory root extract</u>, <u>puffed durum wheat</u>, rice flour, erythritol, palm oil, corn syrup, vegetable glycerin, whole-grain oats, whey protein isolate, <u>whole-grain barley flakes</u>, canola oil, rice starch

Salad Dressing

Ingredients: Canola oil, distilled vinegar, apple cider vinegar, salt, <u>garlic</u>, <u>onion</u>, monosodium glutamate, xanthan gum, beta carotene (color)

Lowfat Plain Probiotic Kefir

Ingredients: <u>Pasteurized organic milk</u>, <u>organic nonfat dry milk</u>, <u>organic inulin</u>, and live cultures, including probiotics: Bifidobacterium lactis BB-12®, L. acidophilus LA-5®, L. casei, L. rhamnosus LB3

Figure 6: Finding FODMAPs on a Food Label

Prior to shopping for food, outline a seven-day menu plan for the week ahead. Fill in all three meals as well as snack ideas, and pair it with your grocery list to ensure you have all the low-FODMAP provisions you need. See the Resources for brand name foods to select at the grocery store.

TABLE 25. LOW-FODMAP, GUT-FRIENDLY GROCERY LIST

| **Grains and grain-based products**

Grains are a good source of gut-microbe-loving fiber, and some provide resistant starch and beta-glucan prebiotics. | Buckwheat, cornmeal, millet, oats, oat bran, polenta, quinoa, rice, slow-leavened wheat or spelt bread bread, sorghum, teff, tortillas, gluten-free or chickpea pasta |

Protein	Soy-based: Firm tofu, tempeh, edamame
We love plant-based legume proteins as they provide oligosaccharide fibers, a key prebiotic fiber for gut health; enjoy these per your tolerance. Animal-based proteins tend to be FODMAP-free, making them easier on the gut, especially during an IBS flare.	Legumes: Canned chickpeas, canned lentils Animal sources: Eggs, lean beef, poultry, fish (including canned tuna), lamb, pork, shellfish
Vegetables *Fiber-rich vegetables help maintain the protective intestinal barrier and can be a great source of prebiotics to support health-promoting gut microbes.*	Arugula, bamboo shoots, bean sprouts, beets (canned or pickled), bell pepper, bok choy, broccoli (florets), cabbage (common and red), capers, carrots, cassava, celeriac, chili pepper, collard greens, corn (cob or canned), cucumber, edamame, eggplant, endive, ginger, green beans, jicama, kale, leek (greens only), lettuce, olives, oyster mushrooms, parsnips, potatoes (white and red skin), pumpkin (canned), radish, rutabaga, scallions (green part only), seaweed, spinach, squash (spaghetti, pattypan, kabocha), sweet potato, Swiss chard, taro root, tomatillos, tomatoes (canned or small amount of fresh), turnip, water chestnuts, watercress, zucchini
Fruits *The brightly colored pigments in fruits tend to be rich in antioxidants and polyphenols; many are prebiotic sources.*	Avocado, bananas, banana chips, blueberries, cantaloupe, clementine oranges, coconut (fresh and dried), cranberries (raw), dragon fruit, guava, honeydew, kiwifruit (gold and green), lemon, lime, orange, papaya, passionfruit, pineapple, plantain, pomegranate arils, raisins, raspberries, rhubarb, starfruit, strawberries

Dairy products and alternatives *These include gut-friendly fermented foods such as yogurt, kefir, and cheeses made with live and active cultures.*	Select low-lactose options if you are sensitive to lactose: lactose-free yogurt, lactose-free kefir, hard and semisoft cheeses such as brie, camembert, colby, cheddar, feta, goat, havarti, mozzarella, Parmesan, pecorino, and Swiss
Healthy fats *The polyphenols in extra-virgin olive oil have been shown to reduce the risk of chronic health conditions. This effect may be due to the favorable prebiotics they provide to the gut microbiome.*	Extra-virgin olive oil, flax oil, avocado oil
Spices *Some preliminary science reveals that certain spices may enhance digestive health via their positive changes on the gut microbiome and metabolism.*	Allspice, black pepper, cardamom, chili powder (without garlic/onion), Chinese five spice, cinnamon, cloves, coriander seeds, cumin, curry powder, mustard seeds, nutmeg, paprika, saffron, star anise, turmeric
Baking supplies *Select suitable whole-grain flours for baking, such as almond flour and oat flour. These boost prebiotics and gut-friendly fats and fibers.*	Almond flour, buckwheat flour, oat flour, gluten-free flour blend that contains whole grains and low-FODMAP ingredients Cocoa powder Dark chocolate morsels Maple syrup Baking powder and baking soda Almond and vanilla extract Pumpkin (canned)

Refrigerated fermented foods *Consuming fermented foods with live cultures is associated with greater gut microbiota diversity, a marker of good gut health.* *Note: Start with small portions of fermented foods to assess tolerance, such as 1/4 cup kvass or kombucha, or 1 tablespoon kimchi or miso. Larger portions of these foods veer into higher FODMAP levels.*	Kvass, kombucha, kimchi, miso, tempeh
Nuts and seeds *These are great sources of magnesium and healthy fats to support your gut and heart.*	Nuts: Almonds, Brazil nuts, chestnuts, macadamia nuts, peanuts, pecans, tiger nuts, walnuts Seeds: Chia, flax, hemp, poppy, pumpkin, sesame, sunflower
Snacks *You and your gut microbes should enjoy a nice prebiotic treat!*	Dark chocolate Popcorn Trail mix made with low-FODMAP portions of nuts, seeds, dried fruits* *Most dried fruits are high-FODMAP; limit consumption to 1 tablespoon raisins or dried cranberries

Well, there you have it—the many details of executing a gut- and IBS-friendly meal plan. If you feel a bit overwhelmed, that's perfectly normal! We've packed a lot of detail into this chapter. Sit back, relax, and give yourself and your brain time to digest the material. When you are ready, start drafting ideas for yummy meals and snacks that appeal to you. From there, create a grocery list to ensure that you purchase what you need. Don't expect to be a perfectionist when you begin a diet change—that is never the goal. Simply explore the impact of foods on your gut and, yes, even on your mental health. Think of making dietary changes as an experiment to gain a better understanding of what foods work for you and your sensitive gut.

CHAPTER 7

MAKING SANE FOOD CHOICES IN A FOOD-FEAR AND WEIGHT-OBSESSED CULTURE

There is a fine line between making lifestyle and diet changes that benefit your well-being and taking drastic measures that are counterproductive and degrade both mental and physical health. Reasonable efforts to nourish your body, like taking extra time to prepare meals from scratch, are admirable. Likewise, limiting certain foods for good IBS symptom control is very appropriate. For example, avoiding lactose, the milk sugar contained in many dairy products, due to repeated episodes of lactose intolerance (pain associated with consuming lactose) is normal. Limiting onions because they trigger painful gas is a natural and suitable response.

The problem occurs when attempts to eat for health or gut symptom control become too extreme, leading to severe over-restriction of food. Signs of this include making excessive rules around food and having an obsession with diet. There is a tipping point of diminished return. Relentless efforts to control digestive symptoms with a highly restricted diet may place you at risk for malnutrition or developing an eating disorder.

Even though hearing these words can make some people feel self-protective and that their lived experience is not fully understood, it is vital to check in with yourself or your health-care team to be sure you are not going down a dangerous path. Unhealthy weight loss can lead to—or worsen—digestive problems. It can have negative effects on gut motility, a decline in muscle function in the pelvic floor that normally allows for ease of bowel movements, and can trigger undesirable changes to the gut microbiome (the microbes that reside naturally in the intestine). Eating disorders come with even more severe risks; in fact, anorexia nervosa has the highest mortality rate of any psychiatric disorder.

Every day in our clinics we treat individuals with IBS who have an impaired relationship with food along with their gut symptoms. We see you, and we completely understand how difficult it can be to navigate a digestive condition that can be worsened by doing something you have to do to survive: eat! But we know that you deserve a healthier path.

It's very possible, too, that some of this information does not pertain to your clinical situation. Still, we address the topic in this book because experience has shown us that some individuals with IBS go down a road with diet that does not serve them and places them at great mental and physical health risk.

UNDERSTANDING VIGILANCE VERSUS HYPERVIGILANCE WITH DIET

Does the mere thought of eating something get you anxious? When you suffer from gut distress, the threat of abdominal pain from eating can naturally prompt you to be vigilant about your diet. And as we saw with the elimination diet (in Chapter 5), identifying and steering clear of known food triggers can help you avoid unnecessary pain and digestive problems. However, it's important to avoid taking caution to an overzealous level. Hypervigilance with diet occurs when one feels a constant threat related to eating any or most foods. It's stressful, anxiety producing, and downright exhausting for the body and mind to maintain this level of caution with every bite. When one is engaged in hypervigilance surrounding diet choices, even safe food environments feel threatening. The mind is perpetually and overly engaged in every single food decision. We sometimes see this behaviorally when a person has been tracking every bite of food they consume for months or even years. Hypervigilance is part of the body's fight-or-flight response. If you are on high alert about any food-related decision, it can lead to feeling restless and irritable, and can interfere with sleep and well-being.

Research has shown that some people with IBS restrict foods to a greater extent than is necessary to manage this complex disorder. Being hypervigilant with diet starts to resemble disordered eating, the preliminary diagnosis that can precede an eating disorder. A registered dietitian with expertise in GI disorders can guide you with a gentle diet expansion to help keep your symptoms at bay while you enjoy a more liberal and delicious diet.

DISORDERED EATING RISKS IN IBS

It is estimated that about one-quarter of people living with a GI condition are at risk for disordered eating. In fact, 43 percent of IBS patients will skip a meal, even when hungry, to control GI symptoms. Disordered eating describes an eating pattern associated with skipping meals, limiting many foods, or following a highly restrictive diet that is not medically necessary.

Warning signs that your diet might be heading toward a disordered eating pattern include the following:

- You do not eat three meals a day.
- You skip snacks, even when hungry.
- You avoid dining out with family or friends.

A true eating disorder may be emerging if:

- Your eating behaviors are severe and restrictive, causing you to limit yourself to only a handful of different food options.
- Your motivation for restriction includes significant fear of gaining weight.
- You experience distressing thoughts and emotions related to your relationship with eating and your body image.
- Your diet is affecting your ability to nourish your body properly, leading to negative psychological and physical effects (amping up anxiety and weight loss).

If you or your loved ones are concerned about your eating behaviors, a licensed medical doctor or psychologist would be best suited to make an official eating disorder diagnosis after careful evaluation. The sooner you get help with disordered eating or an eating disorder, the better your likelihood of making a full recovery. We want you to know that the body is incredibly resilient. Past eating behaviors can in fact have long-term consequences, but the body can also heal!

EATING DISORDERS: WHAT ARE THEY AND HOW CAN THEY AFFECT THE GUT?

Unfortunately, the prevalence of disordered eating is growing exponentially. Like IBS, it's more common in women than men.

However, there is an unfolding story regarding prevalence of eating disorders and gender. At this time, men account for only 10 percent of research participants with anorexia nervosa or bulimia nervosa. There are also interesting gender differences: men tend to be concerned with attaining muscle, while women are more concerned with being thin. We suspect that prevalence rates for men will increase as screening measures improve across gender and more men seek treatment.

A recent study revealed that eating disorders more than doubled between the time period of 2000–2006 and the time period of 2013–2018. The main eating disorders include anorexia nervosa, bulimia nervosa, and binge-eating disorder. (These are described with detailed diagnostic criteria in the fifth edition of the *Diagnostic and Statistical Manual of Mental Disorders*, or *DSM-5*, a publication from the American Psychiatric Association.)

Anorexia nervosa presents with excessive dieting that leads to severe weight loss. It is associated with an extreme fear of becoming fat. Bulimia nervosa occurs with loss of control over one's eating, followed by inappropriate behaviors such as self-induced vomiting or laxative abuse to avoid weight gain. Binge-eating disorder is more severe than simply overeating. The individual experiences a sense of losing control over their eating. They may also feel guilt or shame, binge alone or in secret, or eat even when not hungry.

Having a past history of an eating disorder increases one's risk of chronic GI symptoms. It's estimated that up to 52 percent of individuals with eating disorders fit the criteria for IBS. The consequences of eating disorder behavior—whether it be malnutrition, purging, or laxative abuse—have a multitude of implications for GI symptoms. Severe malnourishment and related muscle loss can lead to malfunction of the pelvic floor muscles, interfering with normal bowel movements. Constipation with retainment of stool in the colon can lead to the problematic sensation of bloating (the sensation of fullness), common in up to 90 percent of those with IBS. Poor nutrition can delay stomach emptying, leading to the GI symptoms of nausea, postmeal fullness, bloating, and abdominal distention (an increase in abdominal circumference).

Eating disorders are serious mental health conditions that can be deadly. Individuals with anorexia nervosa who have received inpatient treatment (care provided in a hospital or treatment facility where the patient is admitted for days at a time) have a risk of death that is more than five times greater in a given year than that of healthy individuals. For those with bulimia nervosa treated in an outpatient setting (care that doesn't require an overnight stay in a hospital or treatment facility), risk of death is twice that of healthy individuals without this condition.

Because of these significant health concerns, some individuals with IBS who are at greater risk for eating disorders should consider treatment options that do not necessitate major diet change. Effective IBS treatments include supportive nutrition or behavioral therapies (see Chapters 2, 3, and 4). If you are concerned about your eating habits and health, we recommend meeting with a specialist in disordered eating (see Resources to locate a provider). Or you can consider other treatments based on specific IBS symptoms that are troubling you (see Chapter 9). Of course, always discuss any concerns with your health-care provider.

BEYOND PICKY EATING: AVOIDANT/ RESTRICTIVE FOOD INTAKE DISORDER

Avoidant or restrictive eating occurs along a spectrum that many patients with GI conditions, including IBS, may fit into. Avoidant/restrictive food intake disorder (ARFID) is characterized by extreme "pickiness" in which food restriction occurs to an unsafe degree. Historically, this diagnosis was most common in children, but recently it has become an expanding area of research in adults with GI conditions.

ARFID is more complicated than just being a very picky eater. Food restriction in ARFID is driven by a lack of interest in eating or food (e.g., forgetting to eat or feeling full quickly and therefore stopping a meal), avoidance based on the sensory characteristics of food (the taste, smell, or sight), or concern about adverse consequences of eating (e.g., stomach pain, nausea, vomiting). In GI patients, adverse consequences may include pain with eating or bowel urgency. ARFID commonly co-occurs with anxiety. Food restriction in ARFID differs from what is typical of other eating disorders, however, in that body image or fear of weight gain is not the motivating factor.

According to the *DSM-5*, ARFID is diagnosed when:

- An eating or feeding disturbance (e.g., apparent lack of interest in eating or food; avoidance based on the sensory characteristics of food; concern about aversive consequences of eating) is present as manifested by persistent failure to meet appropriate nutritional or energy needs associated with one (or more) of the following:
  - Significant weight loss (or failure to achieve expected weight gain or faltering growth in children);
  - Significant nutritional deficiency;
  - Dependence on enteral feeding or oral nutritional supplements; or
  - Marked interference with psychosocial functioning.

- The disturbance is not better explained by lack of available food or by a culturally sanctioned practice.
- The eating disturbance does not occur exclusively during the course of anorexia nervosa or bulimia nervosa, and there is no evidence of a disturbance in the way in which one's body weight or shape is experienced.

- The eating disturbance is not attributable to a concurrent medical condition or not better explained by another mental disorder. When the eating disturbance occurs in the context of another condition or disorder, the severity of the eating disturbance exceeds that routinely associated with the condition or disorder and warrants additional clinical attention.

Preliminary research reveals that ARFID risk is higher in people living with GI disorders. As you can imagine, assessment for ARFID is a bit challenging, as food fears are common when eating is a trigger for GI distress. Since food-related symptoms are common to GI conditions, reasonable dietary restrictions are appropriate. That being said, scientists are seeing ARFID-like behaviors in adults with a variety of GI conditions, such as celiac disease, eosinophilic esophagitis, IBS, and inflammatory bowel disease. When fear of food leads to deterioration of mental health or nutritional deficiencies, then an ARFID diagnosis should be considered. For guidance in finding an expert to help, see Finding an Eating Disorder Specialist in the Resources (page 327).

WHEN HEALTHY EATING GOES TOO FAR: ORTHOREXIA

- Has skipping social events and avoiding dining out with friends become your new normal?
- Have family members or trusted friends expressed concern over your extreme food rules?
- Are you frequently worried about the nutritional value of a food? Do you obsessively examine food labels?
- Do you continuously think about meal planning, food preparation, and eating, to a point that it feels exhausting?

- Do you categorize foods as "good" or "bad" and experience guilt if you eat a "bad" food?

If you answered yes to any of the above, you may want to talk with a health-care provider about orthorexia. This is another condition we see in our clinical GI practices. Orthorexia nervosa is described as having a pathological obsession with healthy eating. While choosing to eat nourishing foods can of course be part of a healthy lifestyle (we love healthy food too!), orthorexia takes it to an unhealthy level. This unsafe focus on foods may impair quality of life and mental well-being. As food choices become obsessive, sufferers find themselves limiting once-joyful social engagements that include food, such as family meals or going to a restaurant with friends. Because the research on this condition is somewhat limited, orthorexia nervosa does not have its own classification in the *DSM-5*; still, it remains of concern with health professionals due to its potential risks to the body and the mind.

Studies have revealed that people following a diet for digestive issues or food intolerances are at a higher risk for orthorexia. It has been hard to capture true prevalence rates of orthorexia, with wide ranges across countries and populations. Individuals who have diagnosed themselves with orthorexia report that managing a chronic disease contributed to their unhealthy, all-encompassing, or extensive obsession with healthy eating. Orthorexia sets the stage for those with perfectionistic tendencies, commonly found in this disorder, to flex their so-called type A qualities of control and structure around their food and nutrition. This can become a slippery slope because aspects of orthorexia can easily be masked by an outward appearance of "health." If the quest for healthy foods becomes a stressor in your life, or social engagements are fraught with a lack of enjoyment of food, or loved ones are commenting on your preoccupation with "health," it is time to speak with your health-care provider about these issues.

INTUITIVE EATING: AN INTRODUCTION

One of our favorite approaches to fostering a good relationship with food is a model of eating called Intuitive Eating. It is associated with improving psychological health and promoting a positive attitude toward food and the body.

Intuitive Eating (IE) is not a diet. Rather, it is a path to guide you toward a healthy and nurturing relationship with food and your body. The IE philosophy embodies ten key principles that encourage you to tune in to how food makes you feel, physically and emotionally. If you need to be on a medically therapeutic diet (such as a low-FODMAP diet), you can still embrace the principles of IE. The IE approach is associated with higher self-esteem, fewer depressive symptoms, improved body satisfaction, and less disordered-eating behavior. We believe it is an ideal lens through which to view healthy eating in IBS.

IE helps you listen more intently to your internal cues (messages from your gut and mind) and pay less attention to external cues (e.g., messages you find online, such as fear-based food rules). The truth is, we are constantly bombarded with media screaming at us to avoid "toxic" foods or to be thinner. Ultimately, one of the goals of IE is to help you reconnect to the pleasure of eating delicious foods—no guilt allowed!

Evelyn Tribole and Elyse Resch, two registered dietitians, developed the IE framework. It has been researched in nearly two hundred studies, showing many health benefits. Years ago, Kate interviewed Evelyn Tribole about Intuitive Eating. Something she said really resonated with Kate, and we think it is very fitting for anyone living with GI symptoms: "Your choices should come from a desire to feel good inside your body rather than a desire to attempt to control your body."

One of the foundations of Intuitive Eating is *interoceptive awareness*. Interoceptive awareness involves tuning in to your body's messages to help you meet your biological and psychological needs.

Emotions, although they may be conjured up in our brain, often result in physical sensations. We experience this, for example, when feeling nervous is accompanied by a pounding heart and an urgent need to get to a bathroom. Interoceptive awareness is a necessary skill to identify the appropriate coping skills to manage the GI stress cycle (see Chapter 2). Without an interruption (which we like to call a cycle breaker), the cycle produces GI sensations → anxious thoughts (about food, stress, symptoms) → anxious emotions → uncomfortable sensations in the body → GI distress. The key to interoceptive awareness is to connect with your body, hear what it's telling you, and gently address what you might need.

INTEROCEPTIVE AWARENESS IN REAL LIFE

What you *don't* need: obsessive awareness of every abdominal twinge, gas bubble, or change in bowel movement.

What you *do* need: to allow your body to gently signal when:

- It needs more food.
- The recognition that eating onions (for example) repeatedly gives you painful gas. Accordingly, you decide to adjust your intake to the extent possible.
- You find yourself stressed out, experiencing a rapid heart rate and shoulder tension. You take note and respond by breathing deeply to settle your body.

This self-connection can go hand in hand with the IE principles when your digestive tract is stressed. Now let's take a look at the ten IE self-care principles. This approach involves applying all ten. It's important that you don't select just one to incorporate into your lifestyle; they are meant to be incorporated together. For more in-depth learning, see the Resources under Intuitive Eating (page 328).

Principle 1: Reject the Diet Mentality

Avoid falling for the false promises of "diet culture," which encourages quick weight loss (that is deemed to fail). These narratives—often found in the media and online—tend to perpetuate body shame and fat phobia. Another hotbed for snake oil and pseudoscience! Quick-fix diets rarely work for long-term weight management, and in the end they lead to the dieter feeling shame for not maintaining the weight loss.

Take a moment to look around you. Can you spot diet culture? It's everywhere—on your favorite podcasts, in magazines sitting on your coffee table, in your social media feeds, or even when simply talking with your friends or family—and it can be harmful! When you become aware of these sneaky diet messages and promises, you will become adept at finding them. When you read or listen to content that discusses cleanses, describes fast weight-loss plans, or displays an individual's before and after photos following an extreme diet regimen, how does it make you feel? You may find that these messages have become ingrained. What do you say to yourself if your freshly washed jeans are tight? Do you put too much energy throughout your day into thinking about your weight? Do the people you engage with constantly talk about food and dieting? Recognizing diet culture and putting up a boundary against it in your life can be freeing.

BRAIN BITE: TALKING ABOUT EATING

Setting boundaries around how we talk about food may not come naturally, especially across generations. But the language we use about food and our body is important within families. Here are some ways to reject diet culture around the family dinner table and beyond:

- Don't micromanage portions or eating habits. Do instead encourage listening to one's body for hunger cues.
- Do treat all foods as neutral. (Reject the idea of "good" or "bad" foods.)
- Do honor diverse bodies. Different bodies are beautiful.
- Don't compliment weight loss. (Not all weight loss is intentional and may be due to sickness.)
- Do have open conversations about all aspects of health, not just eating (moving your body, relaxing your body, enjoying nature, laughing, and having fun).

Principle 2: Honor Your Hunger

Learn how to recognize your body's hunger cues. When your body sends hunger signals, you simply honor them. Unfortunately, many people with GI conditions skip meals, even when hungry! Ignoring our body's cues can lead to low blood sugar, irritability, and exhaustion. And underfueling the body also backfires, as it later triggers overeating, which can in turn prompt GI symptoms. The goal is to rebuild trust in your body's hunger messages. Learn to honor the first sign of hunger that your body sends you.

Principle 3: Make Peace with Food

Prohibiting foods can lead to food obsession or desire. This principle takes on a bit more complexity when you are dealing with a GI condition in which food can trigger symptoms. The goal here is to understand the "why" behind your food choices. Explore whether you choose to avoid a food due to a specific food rule, or truly because the food repeatedly prompts pain. Attempting to be on the "perfect gut-friendly diet" can lead to deprivation, then guilt and shame when you veer off the diet. Give yourself unconditional permission to eat. Food should never go hand in hand with shame and guilt. Make peace with your nutrition plan—make it sustainable, realistic, and enjoyable!

Principle 4: Challenge the Inner Food Police

We all have an internal voice that speaks to us. Don't allow your inner food critic to ever make you feel guilty about a food choice. Again, guilt and shame have no place with eating.

Principle 5: Discover the Satisfaction Factor

How can you make eating more satisfying? The book *Intuitive Eating* sums up this concept very well: "When you eat what you really want, in an environment that is inviting, the pleasure you derive will be a powerful force in helping you feel satisfied and content." So if you eat a bowl of bone broth because you heard it was good for you, and you absolutely are grossed out by the taste and experience, consider this permission to eat something else. Yes, you deserve to enjoy and feel satisfied with what you eat!

Principle 6: Feel Your Fullness

Trust not only the signals of hunger but also the signals of fullness. Check in midmeal to be aware of the taste of your meal and your level of fullness. Stop if you are full, and keep eating if you are not satiated. The clean-plate club has closed its doors. You aren't required to finish every piece of food on your plate.

Principle 7: Cope with Your Emotions with Kindness

While food can affect our mood, it should not be the sole vice for anxiety, loneliness, boredom, or anger. It is important to deal with the source of your feelings and to develop a variety of coping mechanisms.

Principle 8: Respect Your Body

People come in all different shapes and sizes. Learn to accept your genetic makeup, and treat your body with dignity, whatever your size. P.S. Don't use magazine cover photos for comparison; they are highly doctored images.

Principle 9: Movement: Feel the Difference

Engage in the joy of movement instead of viewing exercise as a means to burn calories. Exercise should help you feel energized.

Principle 10: Honor Your Health with Gentle Nutrition

Look at the big picture of what you are eating to honor your health goals. Push past the expectation of having the "perfect diet," and instead view your overall diet pattern as one that is nourishing and nurturing—and joyful too. Treats are welcome here!

BEWARE OF THE SLIPPERY SLOPE OF SOCIAL MEDIA

Back to the internet for a minute. Whether it's the recommendation to give yourself an "internal shower" via a "special chia seed drink," or advice to get probiotics from any fermented food, please know that misinformation about gut-health topics is rampant on social media. We do love the ease of finding a delicious recipe online, but as a source of health advice, social media channels should be regarded warily. Anyone can call themselves a gut-health coach or a holistic nutritionist. That's right, anyone—no credentials needed. We are inundated with health messages from nonprofessional "influencers" on every platform, and it may come as no surprise that many of their popular topics fuel food fear.

These social media messages may prompt you to question every bite you take. How can you sort through the good, bad, and ugly that's out there? For starters, avoid sites and content creators that use terms like "toxic foods," "supplement regimens," "colon cleanses," or "quick-fix" diet solutions. There is often zero science to substantiate their claims.

Social media also exploits celebrities and television doctors who endorse a wide range of potentially dangerous fad diets or supplements, or manipulate or oversimplify the science regarding digestive health and treatments. They do this for one reason: money. Curated messages often suggest highly restrictive diets to cure or "get at the root" of your digestive condition, and again, these claims are almost always based on little scientific fact. To make their recommendations more credible, they may include a "scientific" reference that doesn't hold up to scrutiny—for example, an outdated animal study that may not reflect the impact of their recommendation on an actual human body. (Just a friendly reminder: we are not mice!) If a recommendation piques your interest, run it by your health professional before you give it a go.

GUT GAME CHANGER: IGNORE THESE FEAR-BASED IBS SOCIAL MEDIA MESSAGES

- Any post on leaky gut *syndrome* (there is no such thing)
- Promises to get to "the root cause of IBS" (if we knew how to get to the root cause of IBS, there would not be any IBS)
- Encouragement to use colonics (colonics are not science-based and can be risky)
- Before and after photos of someone's stomach, which encourages body shame (and mostly shows the abs of thin women); don't forget that many of the photos online have been digitally enhanced
- Encouragement to use juicing as a cure (juice can be full of IBS triggers—not a good general tip)

Unfortunately, these messages get through in all the wrong ways. A survey study of about eighteen hundred young adults found that those who utilized social media the most frequently—including Instagram, Facebook, X (formerly known as Twitter), Google+, You-Tube, LinkedIn, Pinterest, Tumblr, Vine, Snapchat, and Reddit—had significantly greater likelihood of experiencing eating concerns. Even though body sizes globally are growing, likely due to several environmental factors, the media still consistently showcases smaller women's bodies—a clear disconnect from normal life and the beauty of body diversity.

The greater the discrepancy between one's current weight and desired weight, the greater the risk of eating disorder behavior. One study evaluated the impact of a television series that celebrated thinness and stigmatized obesity in adolescents. The results? Disordered eating behaviors were significantly more prevalent following exposure to the show. To help navigate the truth behind the often fraudulent information online, always seek guidance from your health-care team.

You can let go of fear-based eating and reclaim eating habits that are sustainable for the long run. Craving a crunchy snack? Feel like enjoying a creamy dessert? Listen to, trust, and address the messages your body is sending. Let go of the notion that food is for nutrition alone, and allow food to be joyful, delicious, and fun. Seek help from your health-care team if you find that your diet has become mentally all-consuming, or if you are concerned that you may be developing disordered eating. We will say it again: shame and guilt do not belong at the dinner table (or the breakfast or lunch table, for that matter)! Work with a dietitian or therapist to help remove these feelings from your meals.

Severity of symptoms and perceived food intolerance are key motivating factors to use diet to quell digestive symptoms in IBS.

It follows that strict adherence to diet therapy is appropriate (to a point) for many people in an effort to evaluate whether dietary change can be effective in managing symptoms. But there is a fine line that places an individual at risk for an eating disorder, and it is easy to cross. Further, if you are someone with a history of an eating disorder, talk with your health-care provider about brain-gut behavioral therapies that may effectively manage your IBS symptoms without requiring that you make dietary changes. If you are concerned that your diet interventions may be going too far, reach out to your health-care team. You should never feel like you are walking alone with your IBS, or that your nutrition plan triggers anxiety because of too much focus on food. The science supports a variety of treatment options. Your Dream Team can help you find them.

CHAPTER 8

FEEDING YOUR GUT MICROBIOME

Whats going on in your gut these days? Even more than you may realize! Your colon contains about 70 percent of all the microbes that reside in and on your body. Known as gut microbiota, this tiny world has taken center stage lately among scientists, consumers, and the media, and for good reason. Scientists are just beginning to understand the unique and complicated relationship between the gut microbiome and its human host, and the critical functions it performs for our health.

Our gut microbes stay busy eating the food particles that escape digestion in the small intestine. Turns out these microscopic creatures have a major job to do. They help ensure optimal digestive function, help us harvest energy from the food we eat, and offer defense against invading pathogens by keeping our gut barrier intact. That's not all. They also produce vitamins, neurotransmitters (brain chemicals that regulate our mood), and other important compounds.

It has become evident that the ecosystem in the gut plays a role in IBS and other GI conditions. It does this via several mechanisms, ranging from the balance of the microbes present to, perhaps more importantly, what they are doing. Diet can affect not only a person's IBS symptoms but also the health of their gut microbiome. In this chapter, you'll learn about gut flora in IBS, the role the microbes play in GI symptoms, the potential role of probiotics and fermented foods, what happens when colonic microbes migrate up to the small intestine, and more.

THE GUT MICROBIOME DICTIONARY: FIVE TERMS TO KNOW

Micro-*what*? Before we dive deeper, here are some key terms associated with the gut and the microbes that find their home there.

Gut microbiota: Also known as **gut flora**. The trillions of microorganisms inhabiting the gastrointestinal tract, including bacteria, viruses, archaea, and fungi. The composition of this microbial community is specific to each person.

Gut microbiome: The collection of microorganisms (and their genes) living in the gastrointestinal tract. Think of the gut microbiome as the house, and the microbiota as the individuals living in the house.

Metabolites (collectively, the **metabolome**): The by-products in part produced by the gut microbes. Examples include short-chain fatty acids, such as butyrate, propionate, acetate; gases, such as hydrogen sulfide, methane, hydrogen; vitamins; and secondary bile acids.

Prebiotics: Certain plant fibers and polyphenols (plant compounds such as flavonoids, phenolic acid, and others) that act as food for our gut microbes. Prebiotics improve the balance of these microorganisms. Examples include fructans, found in onion, garlic, beets, and artichokes; galacto-oligosaccharides, found in legumes such as chickpeas, lentils, and soybeans; beta-glucan, found in oats; and phenolic compounds, found in olive oil.

Probiotics: Live microorganisms that when consumed in adequate amounts can offer health benefits. For example, *Bifidobacterium longum* 35624, found in the Align Probiotic supplement.

WHAT CAN GOOD GUT MICROBES DO FOR YOU?

Your gut microbes—mainly bacteria, but also viruses and fungi like yeast and mold—aren't just chilling out in your colon. They serve many important roles for your health.

Protect Against Disease

Microbes help establish a stable intestinal barrier. Think of your gut like the secrets you keep after a weekend in Vegas, and "what happens in Vegas stays in Vegas." The intestinal barrier helps keep microbes and some of the metabolites they create inside the gut, preventing them from traversing the gut and landing in the bloodstream. An imbalance between health-promoting and pathogenic microbes may be one of the mechanisms that increases the "leakiness" of the gut. Rich in the endotoxin LPS (lipopolysaccharides), certain potentially pathogenic microbes appear to damage the gut lining, increasing permeability and inflammation. Simply put, some of the microbes and their metabolites should stay inside the gut and never enter the bloodstream, where they could gain access to other organs and tissues. An abnormal movement of larger bacterial metabolites into the body's systemic circulation has been linked to many disorders, including IBS, inflammatory bowel disease, and diabetes. Microbes are also important in establishing a healthy immune system, helping the body fend off pathogens and infectious diseases.

Digest Your Food

But wait, there's more! Microbes have the capacity to digest food that the human body otherwise cannot. Our bodies produce digestive enzymes in the GI tract to aid digestion and absorption of nutrients, and our gut bacteria harbor even more of these. Lots of gut microbes contain enzymes that allow them to break down plant fibers that normally escape digestion in the small intestine. Interestingly, the specialized digestive enzymes for fiber are microbe specific. For instance, *Bacteroides*, Ruminococcaceae, and *Faecalibarterium prausnitzii* (whoa, that's a mouthful!) contain digestive enzymes that have a greater capacity to digest carbohydrates.

Your gut microbiome is personal to you—some people have microbes with vast digestive enzyme capacity, and others do not. The capacity to digest carbohydrates readily can enhance the amount of gas present in the colon—though this may vary from person to person, as other microbes present in the gut can cross-feed and consume gas. Excess gas can get trapped in the IBS gut, leading to bloating, cramping, and pain.

Make Metabolites

By digesting food for us, the human gut microbiota produces an enormous amount of metabolites, including important compounds for our health. Many carbs that resist digestion in the small intestine (such as plant-based fibers) are fermented by our gut microbes into short-chain fatty acids (SCFAs). These SCFAs include butyrate (which is known to lower colon cancer risk), acetate (which helps regulate weight and blood sugar), and propionate (which is thought to lower blood fat and cholesterol, offering heart-health benefits). Many microbes produce lactate, a short-chain hydroxy-fatty acid, which can be then fermented into SCFAs by microbes. SCFAs are also associated with lowering the risk of IBS and inflammatory bowel disease, and with regulating the nervous and immune systems. Gut microbes can contribute to mood regulation via the neurotransmitters (brain chemicals) they create, such as dopamine, which plays a role in our feelings of pleasure and helps us maintain focus; gamma-aminobutyric acid (GABA), which has a calming effect; and precursors to serotonin, a "feel good" chemical.

Undigested protein that arrives in the colon is broken down by the gut flora. (Although the body is capable of digesting a fair amount of protein, there's a tipping point beyond which excess protein will arrive in the colon intact.) The health benefits of protein metabolism by microbes, however, do not seem to mirror the health benefits provided by their ability to metabolize plant-rich carbs. In fact, too much protein in the diet may contribute to GI symptoms. Passing hydrogen sulfide gas (a stinky fart that smells like rotten eggs) is associated with eating excess protein. In addition, protein fermentation by gut microbes can lead to production of metabolites we don't want, which are associated with intestinal disease—including increasing the risk of "leaky gut" via thinning of the protective mucus layer of the intestinal barrier.

That said, it's important to get enough protein in your diet to maintain muscles and energy and to promote proper immune function. Spread your protein intake throughout the day to ensure best digestion. In general, you don't want to eat more than 2 grams of protein per kilogram of body weight in a day, which equates to about 130 grams of protein for a person who weighs 65 kilograms (140 pounds).

In short, the food you eat seems to help determine what compounds your microbes produce, which, as we'll see, can in turn affect your IBS. While we don't have all the answers about how diet influences the gut microbiome, we can offer some general guidance on diet patterns that offer good IBS symptom control and that also have the potential to improve overall gut health and reduce other chronic health risks.

DIGESTIBLE DETAIL: HOW MUCH PROTEIN ARE YOU EATING?

For your reference, here is the approximate protein content of some commonly consumed foods:

 3 ounces chicken: 24 grams (g) of protein

 1 cup firm tofu: 22 g

 2 eggs: 16 g

 1 cup lactose-free cow's milk: 8 g

 2 tablespoons peanut butter: 8 g

 1/4 cup canned chickpeas: 3.5 g

CHARACTERISTICS OF A HEALTHY GUT MICROBIOME

Your gut microbiome's exact mix of microbes is as unique as your fingerprint, except its makeup can change, for better or worse. The human gut is dominated by four phyla (primary groups) of bacteria: Firmicutes, Bacteroidetes, Actinobacteria, and Proteobacteria. Besides bacteria, other types of microorganisms flourish in the gut, including archaea, fungi (yeast and mold), and viruses. A few specific features appear to be markers of a healthy gut microbiome: its stability, balance, and diversity.

A healthy gut microbiome has a good ratio between health-promoting microbes and potentially pathogenic (disease-causing) ones. A stable gut microbiome is one that can bounce back to its normal state following exposure to stressors such as illness, antibiotic use, or even mental stress. Any of these might temporarily change the gut microbial environment.

Microbiota balance can shift with changes in one's age, diet, geographical location, intake of food supplements and drugs, and even with the seasons. When the balance of microbiota is negatively altered, it can increase risk of infection or disease. Antibiotic use, for instance, can change the gut microbiota balance and can put an individual at risk for *Clostridium difficile* (*C. diff*) infection. This condition can be frustrating to resolve, and in its most severe form is life-threatening.

Additionally, a diverse gut microbiome—one that is enriched with a vast variety of different species and strains—is a general marker of a healthier gut microbiome. A reduction in diversity in a bacterial community appears to affect its ability to recover from stressors, and a lack of diversity is observed in numerous chronic health conditions—including IBS, inflammatory bowel disease, and obesity, to name a few.

GUT GAME CHANGER: ARCHAEA

Another type of microbe that calls the GI tract home is called archaea. Like bacteria, archaea are single-celled organisms, but they differ in chemical composition. *Methanobrevibacter smithii*, the most dominant archaeon in the human gut, is well known for producing methane gas and is associated with constipation.

THE IBS GUT MICROBIOME

Although your gut microbiome is personal to you, there are some common attributes seen in many people diagnosed with IBS. One study found that the microbiome of individuals with IBS had significantly lower alpha diversity (a measure of how diverse the microbes are in a single sample), was enriched with gram-negative bacteria (which tend to be more pathogenic or "unhealthy"), and was associated with a reduction in pathways associated with SCFAs and vitamin synthesis (can't make as many metabolites as the body needs).

Recent studies from Dr. Mark Pimentel's lab at Cedars-Sinai Medical Center in Los Angeles have helped identify different types of microbes in the guts of people living with IBS. They have further shown that depending on the presence of certain microbes, different GI symptoms occur. For instance, the microbe called *Methanobrevibacter smithii* produces methane gas, which can slow intestinal contractility, leading to constipation. The onset of postinfectious IBS reveals how pathogenic microbes related to foodborne illness or gastroenteritis can go on to trigger IBS.

Multiple studies have shown that in most people with IBS, eating FODMAP-containing carbohydrates triggers GI symptoms. A high-FODMAP diet in IBS appears to be associated with negative microbiome changes that appear to occur only in the subset of individuals with IBS who respond favorably to a low-FODMAP diet. In other words, those who fail to find symptom relief on a low-FODMAP diet do not appear to experience the same microbiome changes when consuming a diet rich in FODMAPs. As mentioned, FODMAPs are like fast food for our gut microbes, which ferment them and create gas. The gas stretches the IBS gut, triggering GI symptoms.

Specifically, small human and animal studies have shown a high-FODMAP diet in susceptible IBS patients results in a noted increase in lipopolysaccharides (LPS), a bacterial toxin. The LPS from the microbes then triggers immune cells, namely mast cells, to activate and dump numerous inflammatory chemicals into the gut. This complex interaction leads to pain as well as greater intestine permeability, or "leakiness" of the colon. Needless to say, these effects are detrimental to FODMAP-sensitive people with IBS. For these sufferers, reducing dietary FODMAPs also reduces activation of mast cells and the resultant chemical release, mitigating GI symptoms.

As we gain a better understanding of which microbes are common or uncommon in the microbiome of people with IBS compared to those who don't have it—and further, which metabolites the microbes are making that may cause digestive distress—we will be one step closer to precision medicine and targeted treatments. Since IBS presents differently in each person, it's possible that the microbiome plays an important part in driving symptoms in some patients (but not all). You and your provider will work together to gain insights into your individual triggers and create a treatment plan that works best for you and your sensitive gut.

D IS FOR DYSBIOSIS

Alterations in the gut flora—or more specifically, when there's an imbalance of healthy microbes compared to disease-causing microbes—make for a condition called gut microbial dysbiosis. Dysbiosis has been implicated in IBS and in inflammatory bowel disease, celiac disease, diabetes, heart disease, and some cancers. Furthermore, scientists have discovered that it is associated with neurological conditions such as autism, Parkinson's disease, and multiple sclerosis. Although we know that dysbiosis of the gut plays a role in many cases of IBS, more research is needed to understand what works best to repair it. Fecal microbial transplant, probiotics, prebiotics, and diet change are a few of the strategies being studied.

GUT GAME CHANGER: ARE POOP TRANSPLANTS REALLY A THING?

Ah, the fecal microbial transplant (FMT). This is a process in which donor poop is added to an individual's gut via a medical procedure or via ingestion of specialized capsules in an effort to create a more balanced and favorable gut ecosystem. There is some evidence it works! FMT has garnered attention as a very effective treatment for individuals that experience recurrent *Clostridium difficile* infection, a life-threatening infectious diarrheal condition. In IBS, the data for FMT has been mixed, with some studies showing benefit and others showing no change in gut symptoms. Researchers speculate that FMT may offer benefits in IBS due to changes in gut flora and associated changes in fermentation patterns and production of metabolites such as SCFA. FMT appears to have potential as a treatment, but more definitive research is needed before it can be used in clinical practice.

BRAIN BITE: *C. DIFFICILE* ANXIETY

If you have experienced a C. *difficile* infection (C. *diff*), you surely never want to experience it again. About 25 percent of people who have had C. *diff* once will be diagnosed with it again due to incomplete eradication of the initial infection. Anxiety can afflict patients as they navigate life after a C. *diff* infection. To manage the controllable stressors associated with good gut health, drink plenty of fluids, eat a gut-friendly diet, wash your hands frequently, and speak with your medical team if C. *diff*-related stress is significantly affecting your day-to-day functioning.

WHEN MICROBES MIGRATE NORTH: SMALL INTESTINAL BACTERIAL OVERGROWTH

Small intestinal bacterial overgrowth (SIBO) refers to an abnormal condition in which bacteria are present in the small intestine in excessive amounts, causing GI distress. Typically, the small intestine does not contain many bacteria. SIBO is an indicator of dysbiosis and is common in IBS. SIBO and IBS share many symptoms, including abdominal pain, distention, diarrhea, and bloating.

The microbes involved in this condition are those typically found in the colon (the first part of the large intestine), mostly potentially pathogenic species known to create gas. There is some controversy about how often SIBO occurs in conjunction with IBS as the testing methods are imperfect. While some sources report a prevalence of SIBO in IBS as high as 70 percent, a recent meta-analysis reported a 37 percent prevalence, with a higher risk for those with IBS-D.

Excessive bacteria in the small intestine can wreak havoc. They ferment carbs in the small intestine, leading to copious gas and bloating, and have been shown to inactivate bile acids and slow movement in the small intestine. Bile acids are important for helping the body digest fats, so inactivated bile acids can lead to fat malabsorption. Key signs of fat malabsorption include passing stools that are lighter in color, often foul smelling, and difficult to flush. Interestingly, since gut microbes produce the B vitamin folate, some people with SIBO will produce a high level of this vitamin in their blood, which may provide a clue that SIBO is occurring.

What Causes SIBO?

When the motility or immune function of the gut is altered, or the pH is changed (making the gut less acidic), microbes have a better chance of overgrowing. Increased risk for SIBO occurs with:

- Motility disorders of the intestine, such as IBS and colonic inertia (when the colon fails to move properly)
- Dysfunction of intestinal nerves or muscles (which may be caused by exposure to foodborne pathogens, such as in post-infectious IBS)

- Autoimmune or immune-mediated diseases that can impair gut movement (such as diabetes, scleroderma, or hypothyroidism)
- Gut inflammation, such as in untreated celiac disease, inflammatory bowel disease, or small intestinal diverticula (a diverticula is a small, bulging, pouch-like pocket in the gut lining that can become inflamed)

Diagnosing SIBO

SIBO can be diagnosed by either a culture or a breath test. Using a culture from a sample from your small intestine, a positive test would show $\geq 10^3$ colony-forming units (CFUs) per milliliter of aspirate, representing a larger than normal number of bacteria in the small bowel.

Alternatively, and at present, the more common test in clinical practice is a hydrogen lactulose or glucose breath test. The individual is given glucose or lactulose (types of sugar), after which the breath is sampled about every half hour for up to ninety minutes. The gas collected from the breath—hydrogen, hydrogen sulfide, or methane—is solely produced by the microbes in the gut. If there is an overgrowth of microbes in the small intestine, they will feed on the sugar and create larger than normal quantities of gas. According to guidelines from the American College of Gastroenterology, a positive SIBO breath test is a measurement of 20 parts per million (PPM) of hydrogen above the baseline amount during the first ninety minutes, and/or a methane gas level of ≥ 10 PPM. The level of hydrogen sulfide (H_2S) gas that would represent a positive test needs a bit more scientific study, but an increase of ≥ 5 PPM H_2S is considered excessive and is associated with diarrhea and abdominal pain. Trio-Smart is the only commercial test that measures H_2S levels in SIBO; its guidelines note that H_2S levels are considered abnormal if they reach ≥ 3 PPM at any point during the breath test.

Regardless of the exact cutoff for H_2S in a breath test, it appears that at a fairly low level, H_2S can prompt GI symptoms in some people with IBS. While H_2S is associated with benefits such as helping with mucosal repair of the gut and protecting cells from oxidative stress, increased levels of the microbes that produce H_2S have been associated with risk of ulcerative colitis (a form of inflammatory bowel disease) and colon cancer. We have more to learn about this gas, the microbes that make it, and how to treat GI symptoms associated with it.

GUT GAME CHANGER: INTESTINAL METHANOGEN OVERGROWTH (IMO)

Methanobrevibacter smithii (*M. smithii*) appears to be the underlying organism responsible for a positive methane breath test in humans. Because *M. smithii* is an archaeon and can overgrow in areas outside the small intestine, it was recently proposed that the term "intestinal methanogen overgrowth" (IMO) be utilized to describe this condition.

What Problems Does SIBO Cause?

In severe and rare cases, SIBO can damage the intestine. Altered fermentation by the gut microbes, especially via microbes that contain and release LPS, can lead to inflammation in the gut and a condition known as villous atrophy (a flattening of the gut lining). Small intestinal villi are fingerlike projections that aid in the absorption of nutrients, and they are where digestive enzymes are produced in the gut. They expand the gut's surface area for efficient absorption. Villous atrophy can lead to a deficiency in nutrients, particularly vitamin B12, iron, and vitamin D.

How Is SIBO Treated?

The primary treatment for SIBO is antibiotic therapy. Current research has yielded the following recommendations:

- For hydrogen-positive SIBO: 550 milligrams rifaximin three times per day for fourteen days
- For methane-positive SIBO: 550 milligrams rifaximin three times per day with 500 mg neomycin twice per day for ten to fourteen days, though this recommendation is based only on one small study

Other antibiotics, including ciprofloxacin, norfloxacin, and metronidazole, have also been used.

While diets lower in FODMAPs have been observed in clinical practice to reduce troublesome gut symptoms related to SIBO, dietary treatments for this condition have not been formally studied. We believe the diet for SIBO should emphasize nutritional balance to replenish any possible nutrient deficiencies, and perhaps a modification in FODMAPs to aid symptom management.

GUT GAME CHANGER:
BEWARE OF SIBO SNAKE OIL

Caution: Numerous "gut health gurus" promote dietary cures for IBS and SIBO that are highly restrictive and that include the purchase of large amounts of supplements. Be wary of practitioners who promote special "protocols" for SIBO. They are not promoting science but rather are selling SIBO snake oil.

MAXIMIZING GUT HEALTH FOR
THE LONG HAUL IN IBS

In the future, gut-microbiome-targeted approaches to IBS care will likely become standard. However, while it is exciting to consider the idea of individualized treatments for IBS—via analysis of the stool microbiome and personalized probiotics (like many companies now try to sell you)—we are not ready scientifically to recommend this type of approach. The stool microbiome, in fact, provides a very limited snapshot of the flora that lives in the gut. It does not represent the important small bowel dwellers, or those embedded near the gut lining. And although we are gaining an understanding of what a healthy microbiome looks like, more data is needed to guide specific treatments.

Some studies, however, have provided hints about the benefits (and ways) of maximizing the diversity of our gut microbiota. Let's look at the roles played by fermented foods, probiotics, prebiotics, plant-based foods, and other lifestyle factors that have been shown—albeit in mostly small studies—to benefit gut health.

"SHOULD I EAT FERMENTED FOODS?"

Fermented foods are made through the activity of microbes such as yeast and bacteria that are either naturally present on a food source or in the environment (also known as wild fermentation) or are added via live cultures. Wild fermentation is typically how kimchi, fermented soy products, and sauerkraut are made; the addition of a starter culture is how foods like yogurt, sourdough bread, and kefir are created.

Food fermentation has been around for thousands of years as a way to both preserve foods and improve flavor. The process of fermenting foods results in increased acids, which add a tangy flavor while reducing the likelihood of foodborne pathogens, as dangerous microbes typically can't live in a very acidic environment.

So, are fermented foods good for your gut? Probably, although misconceptions abound. A common misconception is that the live and active microbes (also known as cultures) present in traditional fermented foods and beverages such as kombucha, yogurt, sauerkraut, and kimchi are sources of probiotics. But most fermented foods are made from uncharacterized wild microbes that do not meet the required scientific evidence to be probiotics. Some fermented foods do not contain live cultures by the time the food is consumed. They have been killed off during the preparation, such as in sourdough bread (which has been baked) or sauerkraut (which is usually pasteurized). Remember, probiotics by definition are alive. However, just because the microbes in fermented food don't meet the probiotic definition, they may still offer health benefits. See Table 26 for examples of fermented foods that contain live microbes versus those that do not.

TABLE 26. EXAMPLES OF FERMENTED FOODS

Contains live microbes	Fresh kimchi, water- or oil-cured olives, traditional salami, fresh sauerkraut
Does *not* contain live microbes	Tempeh, most wine and beer, sourdough bread, pasteurized sauerkraut

Right now, the scientific evidence on the gut health benefits of fermented foods is limited. Still, fermentation is thought to be beneficial in a few ways—for example, by reducing the phytate content of foods. Phytates are compounds that bind to important minerals in a food, rendering them unavailable to the body. Fermentation results in fewer phytates, allowing for more nutrients in the food to be present for the body to use.

Fermentation can also reduce the lactose content of a food, a bonus for those who experience lactose intolerance. Microbes consume some of the milk sugar during the fermentation process. Science has revealed that drinking kefir aids with lactose absorption as well as with eradication of *H. pylori*, a bacterium associated with stomach and small intestinal ulcers and inflammation.

A small study from Norway found that eating sauerkraut may mitigate IBS symptoms. The researchers looked at both pasteurized sauerkraut (in which the microbes had been killed) and unpasteurized sauerkraut (containing live microbes). Both options offered symptom reduction, but people eating the unpasteurized sauerkraut showed the most improvement.

An important yet small study was conducted by top microbiome experts from Stanford University. It compared a high-fiber diet (40 grams of fiber per day) to a diet rich in fermented foods (about six servings per day) in a group of thirty-six healthy adults. Eighteen participants received a ten-week high-fiber diet, and the other eighteen received a diet rich in fermented foods that contained live and active cultures (e.g., kombucha, kvass, cultured buttermilk, kimchi, fresh sauerkraut, and other fermented vegetables). The scientists measured microbiome metabolites, immune markers, and other things. They found that the diet rich in fermented foods led to an increase in overall gut microbial diversity. The high-fiber diet did not have this effect. Additionally, participants who consumed fermented foods had less immune activation and a reduction in inflammatory markers, including a reduction in interleukin-6, which has been linked to conditions such as rheumatoid arthritis and type 2 diabetes.

This study gained a lot of traction in the medical community. While it is an important and well-designed study, it's crucial to note that it was conducted with a very small number of people (studies using larger groups provide more evidence than small studies), and none of them had IBS. Still, it shows that eating a wide range of fermented foods containing live and active cultures may afford some benefits, including enhanced gut microbial diversity.

Note: If you are FODMAP-sensitive, start by selecting lower-FODMAP fermented foods, and then expand your repertoire of fermented foods based on your tolerance. Table 27 lists a few low- and high-FODMAP fermented foods.

TABLE 27. LOW- AND HIGH-FODMAP FERMENTED FOODS

Low-FODMAP fermented foods	High-FODMAP fermented foods (containing live and active cultures)
Lactose-free yogurt	Buttermilk
Lactose-free kefir	Sauerkraut
Kvass	Kimchi (½ cup)
Kombucha (½ cup)	Kombucha (1 cup)

"SHOULD I TAKE A PROBIOTIC SUPPLEMENT?"

You've probably heard of probiotics—maybe you've even tried taking them. Probiotics are widely touted in the press as an essential gut-health supplement for everyone. But it's not that simple! The reality is, probiotics should be *selected specifically for the symptom or condition you hope to treat, in amounts that have been shown in research to provide such benefit.*

Selecting a probiotic requires an understanding of the microbe down to the strain level (see below for more on strains of microbes). Otherwise, it might offer no help at all—or it could even make your symptoms worse. Here are some key things you should know about probiotics:

- Probiotics are classified by genus, species, and strain—for example, *Lactobacillus* (genus) *plantarum* (species) 299v (strain).

- Different strains of the same species may have different health effects.
- Dose is important! A probiotic consumed at a higher dose may not necessarily afford a greater health benefit than the same probiotic consumed at a lower dose.
- Select a probiotic dose that's been shown in the research to offer the health benefit you are seeking.

The latest science-based guidelines from the American College of Gastroenterology for IBS management recommend against using probiotics for global IBS symptoms. This doesn't mean that a probiotic will not reduce symptoms or offer a health benefit in any individual with IBS. But the existing science is limited. Many probiotics have only been studied in a small number of people (remember, larger studies involving more people provide greater scientific evidence); they use various types and strains of probiotics (studies that show repeatable results using one precise form of treatment have stronger evidence); and the results of most probiotic studies to date have revealed inconsistent improvement for IBS symptoms. That said, some probiotics have been shown to reduce IBS symptoms (see Table 28) and may be worth discussing with your health-care provider. Check out the Resources for additional probiotic options that have shown benefit in IBS.

GUT GAME CHANGER: TRYING A PROBIOTIC

As a rule, one month is typically long enough to judge whether a probiotic is helping your gut symptoms. If you don't find noticeable improvements in your IBS symptoms after the one-month trial, you could try another probiotic, or opt to save your money and stop using them.

TABLE 28. PROBIOTICS WITH SCIENTIFIC EVIDENCE IN IBS

Probiotic name (brand or generic)	Probiotic strains	Dose (CFUs)	Benefit
Align	*Bifidobacterium infantis* 35624	1 billion	Improves abdominal pain, bloating, flatulence, and bowel habit satisfaction in IBS-D and IBS-C
Bio-Kult	*Bacillus subtilis* PXN 21, *Bifidobacterium* spp. (*B. bifidum* PXN 23, *B. breve* PXN 25, *B. infantis* PXN 27, *B. longum* PXN 30), *Lactobacillus* spp. (*L. acidophilus* PXN 35, *L. delbrueckii* spp. *bulgaricus* PXN 39, *L. casei* PXN 37, *L. plantarum* PXN 47, *L. rhamnosus* PXN 54, *L. helveticus* PXN 45, *L. salivarius* PXN 57), *Lactococcus lactis* PXN 63, and *Streptococcus thermophilus* PXN 66	8 billion	Treatment significantly improved the severity of abdominal pain in patients with IBS-D
Lactobacillus plantarum 299v (DSM 9843) (available in several brands)	*Lactobacillus plantarum* 299v (DSM 9843)	10 billion	A four-week treatment provided effective symptom relief in IBS, particularly of abdominal pain and bloating

CFUs: colony-forming units

WHAT ABOUT PREBIOTICS IN IBS?

You can think of prebiotics as food for health-promoting gut microbes. They are found naturally in many plant-based foods. Eating foods rich in prebiotics can provide many benefits.

- Prebiotics may increase the availability of calcium to the body. Calcium absorption is stimulated by the chemical changes and increases in acid from the fermentation of prebiotic dietary fibers by various gut bacteria.
- They may reduce protein fermentation, which is associated with unhealthful metabolite production.
- They can reduce "bad bugs" in the gut. Prebiotics feed the health-promoting microbes, and as the good bacteria grow in number, they leave less food for the pathogenic microbes. Also, many prebiotics are fibers, and as they are fermented by the gut microbes, acid is released into the gut. Many pathogenic microbes cannot live in highly acidic environments, so their numbers are reduced.
- They can help immune function and help maintain the gut barrier.

Here's the rub: most prebiotic food sources contain FODMAPs. Prebiotics are found naturally in foods like onion, garlic, wheat, and beans. Sometimes they are added to a food product in the form of inulin, chicory root extract, or fructo-oligosaccharides. If you are FODMAP-sensitive, don't worry—other foods contain prebiotics too. Oats (cooked or raw) contain the prebiotic beta-glucan. Uncooked oats also provide resistant starch, another potential prebiotic fiber. Check out the recipes for Energy Bites (pages 305 and 306), which include both resistant starch and beta-glucan. Resistant starch is also found in cooked and cooled rice and potatoes. And many colorful plant-based, low-FODMAP foods contain prebiotic polyphenols. Polyphenols can be found in extra-virgin olive oil, kiwifruit, berries, nuts, and even dark chocolate.

Remember to restrict only the FODMAP-containing foods that repeatedly cause you gut distress. If you can tolerate foods with prebiotics, your microbes can use them! You might start with low-FODMAP prebiotic foods if you are FODMAP-sensitive, and then slowly reinstate FODMAP-containing foods up to your personal threshold. You will discover that threshold as you identify your trigger foods during the reintroduction phase of the low-FODMAP elimination diet, outlined in Chapter 5.

Read on for tips to boost your intake of prebiotics on a low-FODMAP diet:

- Consume suitable (or as tolerated) portions of low-FODMAP nuts and seeds such as walnuts, pecans, chia seeds, and pumpkin seeds in at least two meals per day. Nuts and seeds contain small amounts of prebiotics.
- Don't swear off all legumes. Add lower-FODMAP options such as canned chickpeas (¼ cup) or canned lentils (⅓ cup) to a meal or two per day. You can add these to salads or stir them into rice to boost your prebiotic fiber intake.
- Add oats to your daily diet to up your intake of the prebiotic beta-glucan. Add uncooked oats to smoothies or energy bites for resistant starch.
- Add unripe bananas to smoothies, use them as a cereal topping, or include them in your muffin recipes.
- Eat two to three servings per day of fruit that you tolerate. Brightly colored fruits tend to be rich in polyphenols, which offer prebiotic benefits.
- Use extra-virgin olive oil. It contains higher levels of prebiotic polyphenols than most other oils.

WHAT ELSE CAN YOU DO TO IMPROVE YOUR MICROBIOME?

You can follow several more lifestyle measures to benefit your mind, body, and microbes.

1. Add More Kinds of Plants to Your Plate

Like, *way* more. Another study that piqued the interest of gut-loving scientists and nutrition experts came from the American Gut Project, a crowdfunded citizen science project. The study looked at the potential benefit for the gut microbiome of a plant-diverse diet pattern: one that contained thirty *different* plants per week versus one that contained only ten different plants. It found that people who ate the wider assortment of plants had greater diversity in their gut bacteria. Further, their microbes had fewer antibiotic-resistant genes, potentially allowing antibiotics to be more effective.

How can you diversify your plant portfolio for gut health and maintain good symptom control? It's easy! Go slow—an IBS gut tends to be sensitive to drastic diet change. Incorporate an extra fruit or veggie into your normal diet each week, increasing slowly to let your gut adjust.

2. Get More Sleep

There is a strong relationship between sleep disruption and GI disorders. Studies have shown a connection between sleep, immune function, and inflammation. Altered sleep habits have been shown to exacerbate IBS, inflammatory bowel disease, and gastroesoph-ageal reflux disease (GERD). IBS prevalence rates are higher in irregular-shift workers, affecting about 33 percent, compared to a general prevalence in North America of 10–15 percent. And research has shown that rectal hypersensitivity (in other words, a more sensitive colon) is more common in IBS patients who get less sleep. Most studies recommend that people get seven or eight hours of sleep per night.

Looking at the impact of sleep on the gut microbiome, one small study revealed that greater microbiome diversity was associated with better sleep timing and overall habits, while poor sleep was associated with lower diversity.

Here are a few tips from the Centers for Disease Control and Prevention to improve your sleep habits:

- Be consistent. Go to bed at the same time each night, and get up at the same time each morning.
- Keep your bedroom quiet, dark, relaxing, and at a comfortable temperature.
- The only things that should happen in bed are sleep and sex. Keep food, work, and TV watching out of the bedroom.
- Keep your bedroom free of electronic devices.
- Avoid large meals, caffeine, or alcohol before bedtime.
- Get daily movement to physically tire your body, which in turn will help you fall asleep more easily.

If anxiety creeps up at night, try the constructive worry technique described in Chapter 3 on page 91.

3. Keep Moving

"Move it or lose it" is a key phrase when it comes to your microbiome too. Exercise has been shown to increase butyrate (a short-chain fatty acid produced by the gut microbes), which is fuel for colonic cells and reduces colon cancer risk. One study comparing active women and sedentary women found that women who got three hours of exercise per week had increased levels of health-promoting microbes, including *Faecalibacterium prausnitzii*, *Roseburia hominis*, and *Akkermansia muciniphila*. *F. prausnitzii* and *R. hominis* are known butyrate producers. Exercise can also help with symptoms of constipation by boosting intestinal movements, eliminating gas, and prompting a bowel movement.

If you don't yet exercise regularly, remember that you are just one stretch, walk, or pedal stroke away from a healthy routine. It may take some effort and planning to get started, but once you complete an activity that gets your heart rate pumping and sweat dripping, you won't regret it!

WHEN EATING HEALTHY HURTS

There's no question that eating can be a challenge when certain "healthy" foods—fruits, veggies, whole grains such as wheat and rye, and legumes—are also your full-blown IBS trigger foods. A lot of messaging around eating a plant-based, fiber-rich diet streams through various social media platforms bearing the hashtag #guthealth. You might feel overwhelmed and perplexed when you encounter lists of recommended foods that contain FODMAPS and therefore could trigger your IBS.

Remember that diet recommendations are never one-size-fits-all, especially for people who experience a complex condition such as IBS. Soothing a sensitive gut requires slightly different rules (at times personalized for you by a licensed expert, *not* an influencer), and that is okay! Living in pain is never a goal.

Scientific studies have shown that *small* shifts in dietary FODMAPs are more tolerable in IBS patients. Accordingly, we encourage you to expand your diet very gently. Gradually reintroduce foods you may have been avoiding to test your tolerance to different FODMAPs and fibers. Give your sensitive gut and colonic environment extra time to adapt to diet change. And yes, you can still maintain a healthy gut without undertaking drastic diet measures! As you widen your diet's variety to add fermentable foods and plants, let your body guide you. Tuning in to your body with interoceptive awareness (as reviewed in Chapter 7) will help you discover what works for you, as well as what should remain off your plate. The Mind Your Gut Food and Lifestyle Tracker (in the Resources) can be another good tool to help you identify triggers that may be leading to gut symptoms.

If eating certain foods prompts an IBS flare, let your gut settle, and then consider trying a smaller portion of that food. Sometimes you have to push yourself through subtle fear to test a new food, just like you might push yourself when you lift weights or begin a new exercise routine. You might feel a bit tired and like you want to skip those final ten minutes on your bike, but you hang in there, gaining strength and a bit more confidence in your abilities. Moving forward with food reintroductions takes courage, but learning what works for you and your body is imperative for your quality of life and nutrient needs.

DIGESTIBLE DETAIL: TRY, TRY AGAIN

A true food intolerance will occur in a repeatable pattern; it's not just a one-off reaction. If a food reintroduction didn't work the first time, try to repeat it. Sometimes gut reactions are unrelated to the food you ate and are instead due to other things—hello, stress or constipation!

We are in a challenging but exciting time for IBS care. Research and science are evolving to expand our knowledge of the complex microbial world within our bodies and to show us how to partner with the microscopic creatures that reside in that world to enhance our health.

CHAPTER 9

PUTTING IT ALL TOGETHER: SYMPTOM-SPECIFIC INTERVENTIONS

A person's life can change in amazing ways when their treatment team truly hears them and provides a clear plan to guide them toward better health. We want to highlight that sometimes additional testing is needed to gauge the next steps in your treatment plan, and you must truly advocate for yourself with your medical team if symptoms persist. Your medical provider plays an important role in your healing by prescribing medications (and adjusting dosages of those meds) as needed, skillfully performing medical procedures when necessary, and sometimes putting the halt to further testing when your diagnosis is established and a treatment plan that includes behavioral and nutritional interventions is agreed on. The best path forward is one that makes you feel comfortable and fully supported.

This chapter serves as a quick and easy summary of many of the available testing and treatment options for your worst symptoms. Whether you are saddled with constipation, diarrhea, bloating, abdominal pain, anxiety, or depression, we've got a plan for you! As you are well aware by now, managing IBS differs from person to person. The symptom-specific info provided here can help guide further diagnosis if needed, describes medications and supplements to consider, and offers additional targeted ways to soothe the gut (or mind)—from yummy foods to cutting-edge therapies.

BRAIN BITE: YOU DESERVE TRAUMA-INFORMED CARE

Despite high rates of trauma in those with GI disorders, not all medical professionals ask about a history of physical, emotional, verbal, or sexual abuse, or about medical trauma. Given the sensitive nature of most GI testing procedures, we encourage you to talk with your doctor about any concerns you may have related to this aspect of medical care. It is not necessary to disclose the details of a trauma history; however, sharing that you have a history of trauma can aid your trusted provider in creating the safest and most comfortable setting to meet your medical needs. This courageous conversation may allow for a giant leap forward in your healing journey. If you are currently experiencing trauma, we encourage you to seek care with a mental health professional (see the Resources for suggestions).

Not sure which symptoms are the most troublesome for you? You may find that filling out a two-week diary of symptoms, foods, and lifestyle will help you assess your day-to-day GI manifestations. (Don't record for longer than two weeks, though; long-term tracking can lead to unnecessary hypervigilance of symptoms and of bowel habits that can be counterproductive.) A two-week snapshot of your GI symptoms can be helpful to share with your gastroenterologist, dietitian, and psychologist to help connect the dots and facilitate discussion about meaningful changes for your health. We recommend using the Mind Your Gut Food and Lifestyle Tracker found in the Resources.

BRAIN BITE: MEDICATION MANAGEMENT MUST-KNOWS

It is important to know that the first one or two medications you try may not provide complete relief. Don't allow several months to go by with no relief and no changes. Communicate how you feel—side effects, improvements, lack of improvements—to your prescribing provider at around week six. It typically takes six to eight weeks to assess whether a medication is working for you. That said, if you experience severe side effects or intrusive thoughts, contact your provider immediately.

Because this book is a science-based resource, we have included many recommendations that have been studied in large, randomized, controlled trials. We've also included some symptom-management strategies that are based on our vast combined clinical experience and expertise. Note that the following information is not intended to force a standard of care. It is meant to inform your treatment plan in a process of shared decision-making with your health-care provider.

Your comfort and understanding of why a treatment or procedure is (or isn't) right for you are critical on your path to feeling better. Your physician will be able to help you decipher what options make the most sense for your specific clinical presentation. Again, many factors will inform this, including ease of use, availability, cost, science that supports the treatment's efficacy, and, of course, safety. As always, do not self-diagnose or self-treat. Working together with your health-care team is the best way to get you feeling well.

Without further ado, let's consider each of the major IBS symptoms in turn: constipation, diarrhea, abdominal pain, bloating, anxiety, and depression.

CONSTIPATION

When symptoms of constipation are unrelenting, certain diet, behavioral, or lifestyle changes can offer relief. The characteristics of your stool are important, so don't be afraid to look at it closely. Use a Bristol Stool Form Scale (found on page 319 in the Resources) to help you define the shape and consistency of your stools for your conversations with your physician. According to the chart, type 1 stool (separate hard lumps or pellets) and type 2 stool (sausage-shaped and lumpy) that is hard to pass are both typically associated with constipation. If your constipation remains persistent after you've tried some treatments, you and your doctor may consider additional testing.

Constipation: Additional Testing to Consider

A **digital rectal examination** can help identify potential structural disorders (e.g., anal fissures, hemorrhoids, fecal impaction, descending perineum syndrome, anorectal cancer) as well as pelvic floor dyssynergia (a disorder that presents with incoordination of the pelvic floor muscles).

Blood testing to rule out celiac disease. The test will look for markers including tissue transglutaminase immunoglobulin A (tTg IgA) and quantitative IgA levels.

Anorectal physiology testing, undertaken when traditional constipation treatments do not work. This more intensive workup can include one or more of the following tests:

- **Anorectal manometry,** performed in people with symptoms suggestive of a pelvic floor disorder or constipation that has not been responsive to standard medical treatment. It measures the functioning of the anal and rectal muscles that are involved in a normal bowel movement. In the procedure, which takes about thirty minutes, the provider inserts a catheter with a balloon on the end into the anus and rectum. It will provide information regarding the pressures and sensations of the anus and rectum while the patient attempts a bowel movement.

- **Balloon expulsion testing (BET)** evaluates the time required to evacuate a water-filled balloon in a seated position. It may be completed during the same visit as the anorectal manometry.

- **Magnetic resonance (MR) defecography** can assist in identifying pelvic organ prolapse and the bony landmarks, which are necessary to measure pelvic floor motion. It is especially useful for those who are believed to have defecation disorders but have had a normal BET. It is performed while the patient lies face up on an exam table.

- **Sitz-marker test** is the simplest and least expensive of the colonic transit tests. These are typically indicated only after anorectal testing, and after discontinuing medications that can affect colonic transit. For this test, also known as the radio-opaque marker method, an abdominal X-ray is taken

120 hours after twenty or twenty-four markers are ingested each day for three days. Colonic transit is normal if greater than 80 percent of the markers have been passed after 72 hours. If your physician has discussed surgical intervention for your constipation, colonic transit should be reevaluated to confirm a diagnosis of slow-transit constipation. Other types of colonic transit testing, like colon scintigraphy or the motility pH capsule, should be considered when your physician would like to measure gastric emptying or small intestinal transit.

Imaging for high stool burden, a symptom that occurs when the colon is full of extra stool (experienced by some individuals with constipation). A high stool burden may reduce small intestinal movements, contributing to the sensation of bloating in the upper gut. An intestinal ultrasound or simple abdominal X-ray can determine if this is the case, and you and your GI doctor can then discuss options to help eliminate the excess stool, such as partial colonoscopy prep or a different bowel regimen.

A **breath test for intestinal methanogen overgrowth (IMO)** helps check for a surplus of methane-producing microbes. Scientific studies have shown that elevated methane gas in the gut is associated with constipation; reducing the methane gas can reduce the degree of constipation. Treatment includes a course of antibiotics to reduce the microbes associated with excess methane production.

Constipation: Supplements to Consider

If you have not explored fiber supplements to help with constipation relief, here's the scoop: **psyllium husk** has the best evidence that it improves symptoms in IBS-C. This low-fermentable and gel-forming fiber can add bulk to the stool and soften it, making it easier to pass.

You may introduce psyllium fiber into your diet with the following plan: 5 grams fiber daily, divided in two doses, to be taken with fluids and/or meals. Gradually increase at one- to two-week intervals, up to 10–12 grams daily. Response to fiber is individual, though most people should feel a difference in a week or two. After first introducing psyllium husk, you may experience bloating, but this usually subsides after several days. Examples of products that contain psyllium include Metamucil and Konsyl. Individuals with narrowing of the esophagus or obstruction in the GI tract should not take psyllium husk. Given that psyllium can interfere with absorption of some medications, it is advised to take psyllium at least two hours before or after taking medications.

It is also reasonable to try a **probiotic** if science has shown that it benefits constipation. Discontinue use if there is no improvement in symptoms within a month, or try another brand. See Chapter 8 as well as the Resources (page 324) to guide your selection.

Remember to always check with your health-care provider before trying a new supplement.

Medications for Constipation

A variety of medications are available that use different mechanisms to aid constipation. Table 29 contains a comprehensive list of the types of meds often used to treat this condition, with product brands and dosing information. You can use it to guide discussions with your health-care provider. Determining which medication to start with will be informed by the most problematic symptoms you wish to target (be it bowel movement frequency, pain, or global IBS symptoms) and what you have tried in the past. In some instances, to gain insurance approval for a prescription, your physician must document unsuccessful past treatment attempts (e.g., linaclotide was ineffective and therefore the doctor is prescribing tenapanor).

Remember to always check with your health-care provider before trying any new over-the-counter medications.

TABLE 29. CONSTIPATION MEDICATIONS

Medication	Brand-name products	Recommended dose and frequency
Osmotic laxatives *Medications that draw water into the stool, leading to softer, easier-to-pass bowel movements*		
Polyethylene glycol (PEG) laxatives	Miralax, Glycolax	17 g daily
Magnesium hydroxide	Phillips' Milk of Magnesia, Dulcolax Milk of Magnesia	Use as directed on product label
Magnesium oxide	Nature's Bounty brand	Use as directed on product label
Lactulose	Cholac, Constilac, Kristalose	20 g daily
Magnesium citrate	Nature's Bounty brand	Use as directed on product label, starting low at 250 mg, and adjusting with health-care guidance
Stimulant laxatives *Medications that speed up the movement of the bowels by stimulating the nerves that control the muscles lining the digestive tract*		
Bisacodyl	Dulcolax, Correctol	10 mg daily; oral or rectal use
Sennoside	Senokot, Ex-Lax, Perdiem	17.2–34.4 mg daily
Secretagogues *Medications that increase fluid secretion and movement in the GI tract*		
Linaclotide	Linzess	72 µg, 142 µg, or 290 µg daily
Lubiprostone	Amitiza	8–24 µg twice daily
Plecanatide	Trulance	3 mg daily
Tenapanor	Ibsrela	50 mg twice daily
Prokinetics *Medications to promote intestinal motility*		
Prucalopride	Motegrity	2 mg daily

Tricyclic antidepressants may cause constipation; therefore these types of neuromodulators are typically not used when constipation is a predominant symptom. Further, selective serotonin reuptake inhibitors (SSRIs) are not globally recommended in patients with IBS; however, if you have constipation, you and your doctor may explore this option due to the medication's potential to loosen stool.

GUT GAME CHANGER: PUSHERS AND MUSHERS

A simple—and might we say fun—way to think about constipation medications is to classify them as either "pushers" or "mushers." Medications that add water to the colon to soften stool are mushers; these include magnesium citrate, magnesium oxide, polyethylene glycol (Miralax), and sorbitol (found naturally in prunes and kiwifruit). Pushers help move the gut to aid constipation; these include senna, bisacodyl, and even your morning cup of coffee.

Diet Changes for Constipation

Before you significantly restrict your diet to aid with constipation, take note of your eating habits, and aim for three regular meals (and a snack or two) per day, avoiding large meals. Be conscious of what you eat, and exercise moderation in your intake of fat, insoluble fiber, caffeine, and gas-producing foods, such as onions, beans, and whole wheat.

We recommend adding some of the foods listed below to your baseline diet to see if they get things moving:

- **Prunes.** Eating six to twelve prunes per day has been shown to reduce symptoms of constipation. They work via their combination of fiber and sorbitol, a sugar alcohol that pulls water into the gut (and also a FODMAP subtype). Note: If you are FODMAP-sensitive, prunes should be trialed slowly to test your tolerance given that they are rich in sorbitol. We recommend starting with one prune per day; increase as tolerated.

- **Kiwifruit.** Eating two green kiwifruit per day is associated with more frequent bowel movements, increased stool volume, and increased stool softness, making it easier to poop. Check out the Clean-Sweep Take-2 Smoothie recipe (page 290) for a delicious way to enjoy the benefits of this sweet and tangy fruit. Tip: If you buy kiwifruit in bulk, chop them up and freeze them—you'll always have some on hand to add to your favorite smoothie.

- **Flaxseed** provides a source of soluble and insoluble fiber and is known for its lubricating and stool-softening effects. We recommend a starting dose of 1 tablespoon per day. Using ground flaxseed (versus the whole seed) is recommended to maximize digestibility and allow your body better access to the nutrients inside the seed.

- **Adequate fluids.** Aim for 64 ounces of liquid (mostly water) per day. Fluids will boost the laxative effects of fiber.

- **Fiber.** Adult women should consume 21–25 grams of fiber daily, and men should aim for 30–38 grams. As you increase fiber intake, go slowly to allow your body to adjust.

In addition to trying these foods, eat balanced meals, and don't skip! The simple act of eating food stimulates the gastrocolic reflex that prepares your colon for a bowel movement.

GUT GAME CHANGER: FLAXSEED FIX

Did you know that ground flaxseed (also called flaxseed meal) can be used as an egg substitute for baking? If you want to increase your intake of flaxseed, simply mix 1 tablespoon flaxseed meal with 3 tablespoons water to substitute for 1 egg. Allow the blend to sit for a minute or two before adding it to your favorite recipe.

Bowel Habits to Keep You Regular

- Do not ignore messages from your body—when you have the urge to have a bowel movement (BM), listen and go! The longer stool stays in the colon, the more water is pulled out of the stool. Harder stools are more difficult to pass.
- As you wake up in the morning, your gut motility increases. Therefore, thirty to sixty minutes after waking or having breakfast, take a seat on the toilet for a few minutes (no longer than that) if you have yet to have a BM.
- Try a toileting stool, such as the Squatty Potty, which has science to support its use for treating constipation. How does it work? When you're seated on the porcelain throne, placing your feet on a toileting stool will raise your knees above your hips, which opens the angle of the rectal canal for easier pooping. If you don't have a Squatty Potty, you might try to prop your feet on a roll of toilet paper or a stack of books that is tall enough to raise your knees above the hips. (Thank us later!)
- Be aware of the height of your toilet. "Comfort-height" toilets may be marketed as easier to use or more comfortable (because they're taller), but ergonomically they don't assist with the proper pooping position (see page 329).

Psychological and Lifestyle Considerations for Constipation

Mind-Body and Brain-Gut Therapies

Diaphragmatic breathing can be used to calm and massage the digestive system while you're sitting on the toilet attempting to have a bowel movement. This special breathing technique can help you experience a more complete BM by helping the pelvic floor relax. Learn more in Chapter 2, or see page 325 in the Resources for a link and a QR code for a demonstration.

Cognitive behavioral therapy (CBT), **gut-directed hypnotherapy**, **cognitive therapy**, **mindfulness**, and **mindfulness-based stress reduction** may be helpful in the management of constipation symptoms through the development of coping skills, relaxation training, and resilience skills. Complementary activities like exercise, massage, acupuncture, or yoga may also help stimulate colonic movements. You can learn more about various brain-gut therapeutic strategies in Chapters 2 and 3, and about gut-friendly exercise in Chapter 4.

Biofeedback-aided pelvic floor retraining can be considered for those with constipation. Biofeedback is a specialized therapy that incorporates equipment to record or amplify activities of the body (in this case, anorectal or pelvic floor muscle activity) and feed this information back to the patient. Biofeedback has been shown scientifically to help manage and treat chronic constipation. The key to biofeedback is teaching the individual to appropriately coordinate abdominal and pelvic floor motion during a bowel movement. To locate a pelvic floor physical therapist, see the Resources section.

New Therapies

Electroacupuncture is a modern variation on acupuncture that uses electricity to enhance the benefits. (See page 258 for more information on acupuncture.) Electroacupuncture has been shown to improve spontaneity and completeness of a bowel movement in women with severe functional constipation during an eight-week course of treatment; the effect was sustained for twelve weeks after stopping treatment.

Vibrant is a new, nonpharmaceutical treatment for constipation. It's a disposable capsule that one ingests with a glass of water; at a preprogrammed time, it vibrates to gently stimulate the colon mechanically. The timing of the mechanical stimulation is thought to improve natural colonic motility by leveraging the colon's biological clock. Early research by leading constipation experts shows that the capsule is superior to a placebo in improving bowel symptoms as well as quality of life. Use of this intervention requires a consultation with a gastroenterologist. You can learn more about it at www.vibrantgastro.com.

DIARRHEA

As a chronic disorder, IBS-D is associated with frequent episodes of diarrhea, but other conditions may contribute to more persistent diarrhea. In this section, you'll find strategies for treating diarrhea. (Also be sure to check out the IBS-D mimickers in Chapter 10.)

Take a good look at your poop. Doing so may be unpleasant—we know. But the characteristics of your stool are important, so note them, and talk about them with your physician. Referring to the Bristol Stool Form Scale (found on page 319 in the Resources section) can help you describe the shape and consistency of your stools. According to the chart, type 6 stool (mushy consistency with ragged edges) and type 7 stool (liquid consistency with no solid pieces) that are unusually loose are associated with diarrhea. Small, frequent bowel movements with tenesmus (a sensation of needing to go to the bathroom despite an empty bowel) and bleeding may suggest proctitis. Less frequent stools that are larger in volume suggest a small bowel source of diarrhea. Steatorrhea (fatty poop that often floats and is lighter in color) indicates either fat maldigestion or fat malabsorption, which can occur in small intestinal bacterial overgrowth (SIBO) and exocrine pancreatic insufficiency, for instance. These conditions are reviewed in detail in Chapter 10.

GUT GAME CHANGER: CONSTIPATION CAN CAUSE DIARRHEA TOO!

"Overflow" diarrhea can occur in the presence of constipation. This results when stool becomes so hard that it cannot be expelled, and fecal fluid flows around the stool blockage. This type of diarrhea can be confusing; you want to treat it with measures to control the diarrhea, but the primary treatment should aim at constipation.

Diarrhea: Additional Testing to Consider

Endoscopy and colonoscopy. Although these scoping procedures are not needed in every case, they can be useful in the evaluation of chronic diarrhea. Endoscopy is a screening of the inside of the stomach and small intestine. Colonoscopy visually examines the colon via a scope inserted in the rectum. During a colonoscopy, biopsies from the right and left colon are often taken to rule out microscopic colitis and ulcerative colitis. An endoscopy may assess for celiac disease, the presence of *H. pylori* (a bacteria associated with gastric ulcers), or other conditions that may be associated with your symptoms.

Routine blood tests (e.g., complete blood count and metabolic profile) can be used to evaluate fluid and electrolyte balance and assess for nutritional deficiencies and anemia. A high white blood cell count may indicate the presence of infection.

Additional blood tests might be taken to rule out celiac disease, including levels of tissue transglutaminase immunoglobulin A (tTg IgA) and quantitative IgA.

Stool testing may be requested to check fecal calprotectin (or fecal lactoferrin) to rule out inflammatory bowel disease. In some cases, when clinically suspected, ova and parasite testing will be conducted. Bile acid levels may be checked to assess for bile acid malabsorption (more on this condition is provided in Chapter 10).

Breath testing for SIBO or lactose or sucrose malabsorption may be considered, as these conditions are often associated with diarrhea.

- **Glucose or lactulose breath testing** for SIBO will measure the presence and amount of hydrogen and methane gas exhaled from the lungs, which is an indirect measure of the gut microbial metabolism. **Trio-Smart**, a novel at-home test, measures hydrogen, methane, and hydrogen sulfide gas. It can be ordered by your doctor or purchased via the company website (www.triosmartbreath.com). Testing is completed in your home and the results mailed in for analysis.
- **Hydrogen breath testing**, undertaken after ingestion of a lactose substrate, is used to assess whether lactose is digested adequately for possible diagnosis of lactose malabsorption.
- **^{13}C-sucrose breath testing** measures how well sucrose is metabolized for possible diagnosis of sucrose malabsorption or sucrase-isomaltase deficiency.

Imaging studies can reveal anatomic abnormalities such as strictures, fistulas, and diverticula. They can assess the degree and extent of inflammation if diarrhea is associated with inflammatory bowel disease. Imaging is also helpful in diagnosing chronic pancreatitis and locating hormone-secreting tumors.

- **CT enterography** uses computerized tomography imaging and a contrast material to view the small intestine.
- **MR scanning** uses a magnetic field to create detailed images of the organs.
- **X-rays**, among the simplest medical imaging procedures, use electromagnetic radiation. A CT scan builds on this technology by using computers to generate cross-sectional images of the body from a series of X-rays taken from different angles. As you might imagine, CT scans provide more detailed information than plain X-rays.

GUT GAME CHANGER: PARASITIC INFECTIONS

Bacterial and viral gastroenteritis may cause diarrhea that resolves. Protozoan infections, however, such as amoebiasis and giardiasis, can lead to chronic conditions. Typically, testing is only recommended for those who have had potential parasite exposure, for example, if you recently traveled to a developing country, consumed water that may be of poor quality (like drinking river water while camping), or had exposure at a childcare center. See Chapter 10 for more on parasitic infections and testing.

Diarrhea: Supplements to Consider

Psyllium husk may help solidify stool as it forms a gel in the gut that can soak up excess fluids in the colon. We recommend starting with 5 grams daily, divided into two doses, to be taken with fluids and/or meals. Gradually increase at one- to two-week intervals up to 10–12 grams daily.

It is reasonable to try **probiotics** to assess their benefit for diarrheal symptoms. If there is no improvement after a one-month trial, discontinue and try another brand, or opt for other treatment options described in this chapter. See information on probiotics in Chapter 8 and specific brands via websites listed in the Resources.

A trial of **digestive enzymes** may be helpful to reduce diarrhea related specifically to some FODMAP subtypes. For instance, the digestive enzyme lactase may reduce bloating and diarrhea when consuming foods with lactose. Be sure to select a brand that doesn't have FODMAP ingredients if you are FODMAP-sensitive.

A few digestive enzyme supplements are currently marketed to aid FODMAP digestion. Theoretically, these products should offer benefit, and many with IBS say they do help them tolerate FOD-MAP foods better. That said, the scientific evidence for these supplements in individuals with IBS remains limited. Similar to our advice around use of other supplements, if you don't experience benefits by the time you finish one bottle of the product, it is unlikely that buying more will help. Save your money and move on to another intervention!

Remember to always check with your health-care provider before trying a new supplement.

Medications for Diarrhea

Many medications on the market can mitigate diarrhea; these are listed in Table 30. Before trying a new medication, it is important to discuss with your physician the medications you have already tried, your most bothersome symptoms, and what you hope to address (i.e., stool consistency, stool urgency, pain, or global symptoms). This will help guide the meds your physician recommends.

TABLE 30. DIARRHEA MEDICATIONS

Medication	Brand-name products	Recommended dose and frequency
Antispasmodics *Medications that relieve, prevent, or decrease muscle spasms, abdominal pain, and cramping by targeting smooth muscles in the digestive tract*		
Hyoscine butylbromide	Scopolamine	10 mg 3 times per day; may increase up to 20 mg 4 times daily if needed
Dicyclomine	Bentyl	20–40 mg up to 4 times daily
Peppermint oil	IBgard	2 capsules 3 times daily at least 30–90 minutes before each meal, with approximately 240 ml water
Opiates (m-opiate receptor selective) *Medications that slow gut transit, decrease the movement of fluid into the intestines, and increase the amount of fluid reabsorbed in the GI tract*		
Loperamide	Imodium	2–4 mg up to 4 times daily
Diphenoxylate	Lomotil	2.5–5 mg up to 4 times daily
Opium tincture	Laudanum	2–20 drops 4 times daily
Mixed opioid agonists/antagonists *Medications to slow down the motion of the gut*		
Eluxadoline (for those with diarrhea and abdominal pain [IBS-D]; contra-indicated in people without a gallbladder or those who drink more than 3 alcoholic drinks per day)	Viberzi, Truberzi	75 mg or 100 mg 2 times daily

Adrenergic agonists Medications that can relax the bowel and reduce pain sensations		
Clonidine	Catapres	0–0.3 mg 3 times daily
Octreotide	Sandostatin	50–250 mg 3 times daily (subcutaneous injection)
Bile acid sequestrant Medication that prevents bile acids that could trigger diarrhea from acting on the colon		
Colestipol	Colestid	4 g up to 4 times daily
Tricyclic antidepressants/neuromodulators Medications that affect nerve signaling between the GI tract and the brain, which can influence pain signaling and GI function		
Amitriptyline	Elavil	50–100 mg daily
Imipramine	Tofranil	50–100 mg daily
Desipramine	Norpramin	25–100 mg daily
Nortriptyline	Pamelor	25–75 mg daily
Antibiotics Medications that work to stop the growth of bacteria that can cause diarrhea		
Rifaximin	Xifaxin	550 mg 3 times daily for 14 days. Talk with your doctor if you have completed this medication and symptoms persist or have only mildly improved

5-HT3 antagonists Medications that can decrease visceral pain and gastrointestinal motility		
Alosetron (for women with severe symptoms, defined as frequent and severe abdominal pain/discomfort, frequent bowel urgency or fecal incontinence, and/or disability or restriction of daily activities)	Lotronex	0.5 mg 2 times daily for 4 weeks; your doctor may increase dose to 1 mg 2 times daily for another 4 weeks

Diet Changes for Diarrhea

Prior to significantly restricting your diet, take note of your eating habits, and aim for three regular meals (and a snack or two) per day, avoiding large meals. Be conscious of what you eat, and practice moderation in your intake of fat, insoluble fiber, caffeine, and gas-producing foods, such as onions, beans, and whole wheat.

Eating soluble, and less insoluble, fiber is recommended for IBS-D. Insoluble fiber can exacerbate diarrhea, particularly the fiber found in wheat bran, which has been shown to irritate the colon and encourage mucus secretion.

- Incorporate oat-based fiber via rolled oats. Oat flour is an often well-tolerated soluble fiber.
- Fruits and vegetables may be better tolerated when cooked or blended (e.g., made into smoothies or blended soups).
- Cooked green bananas have been shown to offer antidiarrheal effects.
- A trial of the low-FODMAP diet (with dietitian guidance) may be recommended. FODMAP subtypes that pull water

into the gut and may prompt diarrhea include lactose, excess fructose, sorbitol, and mannitol.

Psychological and Lifestyle Considerations for Diarrhea

Mind-Body and Brain-Gut Therapies

Diaphragmatic breathing can be used to calm the digestive system, possibly aiding with the urgency, cramping, and spasming that worsen diarrhea. Learn more in Chapter 2, or go to page 325 for a link and a QR code for a demonstration.

Cognitive behavioral therapy (CBT), **gut-directed hypnotherapy**, **cognitive therapy**, **mindfulness**, and **mindfulness-based stress reduction** may improve diarrhea symptoms by helping you improve coping skills, relaxation, and resilience. Complementing many aspects of brain-gut therapies are healthy lifestyle habits such as physical exercise and calming body work in the form of yoga, meditation, or massage. Learn more about these forms of therapy in Chapters 2, 3, and 4.

Acupuncture is a form of traditional Chinese medicine that should not be overlooked in IBS management. The licensed acupuncturist inserts thin needles into predetermined points in the body. According to the philosophy behind acupuncture, stimulating these points will help restore the balance of one's qi (energy), or the balance between yin and yang, which in turn helps to treat the underlying problem. The needles are sometimes used with the application of heat (moxibustion). While research on acupuncture for patients with IBS-D and abdominal pain is ongoing, it shows promise for reducing symptoms.

New Therapies

Early research at Cedars-Sinai Medical Center shows that **virtual reality** (VR) as a treatment for IBS looks encouraging, especially for symptoms of pain. VR has been shown to help people engage differently with their body, which can change how they react to symptoms and can improve how they cope. You can find VR recommendations in the Resources.

BLOATING

When bloating is your primary symptom, your physician will ask you about alarm signs such as weight loss, rectal bleeding, or anemia. They will also evaluate for possible overlapping disorders of gut-brain interaction—such as functional diarrhea, functional constipation, functional dyspepsia—and for small intestinal bacterial overgrowth. See Figure 7 for factors that may prompt bloating. Talk with your doctor about any recent weight loss or weight gain. Remember, "bloating" refers to the sensation of fullness in your gut, while "abdominal distention" refers to an actual change in your abdominal girth. Using the proper terminology can better inform your provider about what is occurring in your body.

GUT GAME CHANGER: A HIDDEN CAUSE OF BLOATING

What is abdomino-phrenic dyssynergia (APD)? APD describes the failure of the abdominal wall muscle to contract and the diaphragm to relax after a meal. Instead, the anterior abdominal wall relaxes and the diaphragm contracts, redistributing gas, which can lead to the sensation of bloating and visible belly distention. Why this happens in some people is poorly understood. Pelvic floor physical therapy may be warranted to help.

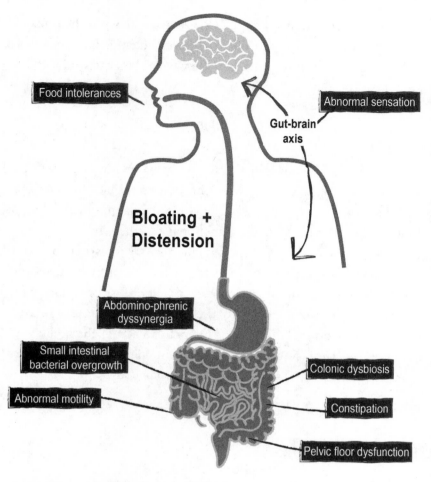

Figure 7. The Complexity of Bloating

Bloating: *Additional Testing to Consider*

- A **physical exam** may reveal signs of bowel obstruction.
- **Rectal and pelvic examinations** should be performed in those who have constipation and bloating.
- **Abdominal ultrasound** or **X-ray** assess for high fecal burden.

Bloating can be a rare sign of malignancy, particularly ovarian cancer. You and your doctor can discuss whether an **ovarian ultrasound** might be indicated to assess for this condition.

Supplements to Consider for Bloating

Although **fiber** appears beneficial in IBS to keep you regular, many people report that it makes bloating worse. If bloating occurs due to a high fecal burden (too much stool in the colon), then clearing the excess stool should help. After stool is cleared, fiber is often better tolerated. See Chapter 5 for gentle fibers to add to your diet that may be well tolerated by your sensitive gut. (Kate often says that adding more fiber to an intestine full of poop is like adding cars to a traffic jam. It doesn't help much!)

The **digestive enzyme alpha galactosidase**, which breaks down the FODMAP subtype galacto-oligosaccharides (see Resources for brands), may help reduce bloating when consuming GOS-containing foods. The dose shown to offer benefit is 300 galactosidase units (GalU).

A trial of the **digestive enzyme lactase** may reduce bloating when consuming foods with lactose (found in dairy). Dosage needs will vary depending on the amount of lactose ingested. Dosing is typically 3,000–9,000 lactase units per meal. (See Resources for brands.)

Peppermint oil taken prior to meals may help reduce abdominal distention and bloating. Peppermint oil relaxes the smooth muscles of the intestine and has antimicrobial effects in the gut. Using an enteric-coated form can reduce the potential side effect of heartburn.

It is reasonable to try **probiotics** for up to one month. Discontinue them if there is no improvement in symptoms, or try another brand. See Chapter 8 and the Resources for a few recommendations.

Remember to always check with your health-care provider before trying a new supplement.

Medications for Bloating

Research has indicated that all licensed drugs for IBS-C are superior to placebo for abdominal bloating. (For a list of many of these to discuss with your doctor, see Table 29, Constipation Medications, on page 245.) Linaclotide has been reported as the most effective. Antispasmodics (such as hyoscyamine and dicyclomine) and neuromodulators (such as desipramine and citalopram) have also shown benefit. Over-the-counter simethicone also offers antibloating properties.

Despite their popularity, evidence is lacking to support the use of activated charcoal and magnesium salts for bloating. Further, Iberogast, an herbal liquid has been shown to improve bloating but is also linked with liver damage. For this reason, we don't recommend it at this time.

Diet Changes for Bloating

Prior to significantly restricting your diet, take note of your eating habits, and aim for three regular meals (and a snack or two) per day, avoiding large meals. Be conscious of what and how you eat (chew your food!), and moderate your intake of fat, insoluble fiber, caffeine, and gas-producing foods, such as onions, beans, and whole wheat.

A low-FODMAP diet can be considered with the guidance of a registered dietitian. Across most of the scientific literature, the low-FODMAP diet has been shown to be particularly helpful for bloating.

Psychological and Lifestyle Considerations for Bloating

Mind-Body and Brain-Gut Therapies

Diaphragmatic breathing can be used to relax abdominal muscles and massage the digestive system. The result may help reduce stress on the body and calm the sensation of bloating. (See Chapter 2 for a description, and page 325 in the Resources for a link and a QR code to access a demonstration.) If diaphragmatic breathing is uncomfortable or worsens the symptom, you can shift to other strategies to activate the body's relaxation response. Physical tension in other parts of the body may worsen bloating; therefore, relaxation interventions offer benefits.

Cognitive behavioral therapy (CBT), **gut-directed hypnotherapy, cognitive therapy, mindfulness**, and **mindfulness-based stress reduction** can provide helpful tools for the management of bloating symptoms. The brain-gut behavioral therapies provide strategies for the development of coping skills and relaxation training if other interventions do not provide adequate relief. Learn more about these forms of therapy in Chapters 2, 3, and 4.

Pelvic Floor Biofeedback or Physical Therapy

Given the fact that the symptoms of constipation and bloating commonly overlap, research supports the use of **pelvic floor biofeedback** to correct defecation difficulties, which in turn can offer significant relief of bloating. Biofeedback with a trained professional can teach you specific strategies for using the abdominal and diaphragmatic muscles.

Abdominal Massage and Light Exercise

Abdominal massage may help move trapped gas toward the rectum for easier elimination. Daily exercise and yoga may help bloating as movement can encourage GI motility. You can learn more about the benefits of moving your body and find a helpful technique for abdominal massage in Chapter 4.

Putting it all together, you can attempt a **simple at-home behavioral practice** to soothe your tummy around mealtime:

1. Sit in a comfortable position, and practice diaphragmatic breathing for five minutes before your meal.
2. While enjoying your meal, chew well, relax, and take your time.

3. At the conclusion of your meal, take five minutes for diaphragmatic breathing. Incorporate gentle abdominal massage or stretching as it feels comfortable.

4. Take a brief walk after mealtime to get fresh air, boost endorphins (especially if there's sunshine!), and generate healthy movement and energy through the body as your feet hit the pavement. Even better, have a friend or family member join you.

ABDOMINAL PAIN

Abdominal pain is a classic IBS symptom, and obviously it's frustrating. (To receive a diagnosis of IBS, abdominal pain must be present in addition to diarrhea, constipation, or both.) This section provides information about testing, supplements, nutrition, and behavioral tips that can help you manage the pain.

A discussion with your health-care provider about the type of pain you are experiencing will help guide potential testing and treatments. While completing a physical exam, your provider can typically identify whether the pain is *abdominal wall pain* (acute, localized—perhaps near an old surgical scar—and described as sharp and extremely tender to the touch) or *visceral abdominal pain* (happens when the nerves are activated; pain can be nonlocalized, vague, and described as pressure, aching, or squeezing).

Abdominal Pain:
Additional Testing to Consider

Carnett's sign is a helpful technique that can be done in a routine visit. The provider will feel your abdomen before and during a contraction of your abdominal muscles. Surprisingly, a positive Carnett's sign—meaning the pain gets worse when the abdominal wall becomes more tense—has a diagnostic accuracy of 97 percent.

Abdominal wall pain may occur with a hernia or nerve entrapment, which may require alternative treatments. A negative Carnett's sign suggests visceral pain.

Abdominal computed tomography (CT) is a noninvasive imaging procedure that shows detailed images of the abdominal organs and structures to provide your doctor with more information about possible injury or diseases of those organs.

Abdominal magnetic resonance imaging (MRI) is another noninvasive procedure that uses powerful magnets and radio waves to produce pictures of the inside of your abdomen without exposure to ionizing radiation (X-rays). During the procedure, you lie down on a narrow table that slides into a large, tunnel-like tube within a scanner. If this sounds like it might provoke anxiety, talk with the technicians. They can offer ways to calm your worries. During an MRI is a great time to practice muscle relaxation and deep breathing.

Upper endoscopy/esophagogastroduodenoscopy (EGD) involves having a flexible tube with a light and camera (endoscope) passed through the mouth, down the throat, and through the esophagus to look at the esophagus, stomach, and upper small intestine. It is typically performed with a level of sedation that makes sense for the patient's comfort level.

In a **colonoscopy**, a flexible scope with a light and camera (a colonoscope) is passed through the rectum to examine and detect abnormalities in the rectum and the entirety of the large intestine. In the United States, almost all colonoscopies are performed with the patient under a level of sedation or anesthesia that prevents them from feeling anything.

Laparoscopy-guided biopsy may be done for women who present with lower abdominal pain or chronic pelvic pain to assess for endometriosis.

Supplements to Consider for Abdominal Pain

Peppermint oil before meals has been shown to reduce global IBS symptoms, which includes pain. We recommend enteric-coated peppermint oil to avoid the potential side effect of heartburn.

Xylose isomerase is an enzyme that can encourage the intestine to convert poorly absorbed fructose (boo!) into well-absorbed glucose (yay!). One study revealed that taking this enzyme helped reduce nausea and abdominal pain in symptomatic individuals who noted malabsorption of fructose on a breath test.

It is reasonable to try **probiotics** for up to one month; after the trial period, discontinue use if there is no improvement in symptoms, or try another brand. See Chapter 8 and the Resources for examples of varieties to try.

Remember to always check with your health-care provider before trying a new supplement.

Medications for Abdominal Pain

While you may be surprised to learn that an antidepressant is recommended for IBS pain management, **tricyclic antidepressants (TCAs)** are the first choice for those with chronic abdominal pain. The initial dose is 10 to 50 mg daily, up to a range of 25 to 150 mg daily. The dose should be increased only if necessary and as tolerated. The dose to treat abdominal pain is typically below what is considered appropriate for the management of psychological conditions such as anxiety and depression. Gastroenterologists tend to be very comfortable prescribing these medications for GI symptoms.

Despite a lack of evidence, **serotonin-norepinephrine reuptake inhibitors (SNRIs)** may be considered for patients with severe refractory abdominal pain. SNRIs may be tolerated better than TCAs because they lack some of the side effects that can occur with TCAs, such as heart palpations, dry skin and mucous membranes, and constipation. When a single antidepressant is not helpful, augmentation therapy, such as multiple antidepressants, or combining an antidepressant with brain-gut behavioral therapy may be suggested. Further, it may be helpful to work with a psychiatrist when utilizing these medications to aid with managing side effects and more complicated medication augmentations.

Antispasmodics (such as hyoscyamine, hyoscine, dicyclomine, and peppermint oil) may be used for abdominal pain. It is important to receive clear directions from your prescribing provider about how and when to take these medications—for example, before or after meals, or daily versus as needed.

For abdominal wall pain, your provider may recommend injection of a **local anesthetic** (such as lidocaine or bupivacaine) with or without a corticosteroid (such as methylprednisolone acetate) at the site of maximal tenderness. Other options, supported by limited evidence, include use of lidocaine patches, heat, and gabapentin.

Diet Changes for Abdominal Pain

Prior to significantly restricting your diet, take note of your eating habits, and aim for three regular meals (and a snack or two) per day, avoiding large meals. Be conscious of what you eat, and exercise moderation in your intake of fat, insoluble fiber, caffeine, and gas-producing foods, such as onions, beans, and whole wheat.

Consider the low-FODMAP diet under the guidance of a registered dietitian, or another individualized nutrition therapy shown to improve symptoms of abdominal pain.

Too much fiber can exacerbate constipation or gas, potentially contributing to pain. A dietitian or other health-care provider can assess your fiber intake and possibly make suggestions to increase fiber, decrease fiber, or change types depending on your presentation. In IBS, a sensitive gut needs slow diet adjustments, especially when it comes to fiber. It's easy to have too much of a good thing!

Psychological and Lifestyle Considerations for Abdominal Pain

Psychological Therapies

If you are suffering with chronic abdominal pain, you know it can really interfere with your overall quality of life—even affect your ability to function day-to-day. In fact, the prevalence of depression in abdominal pain patients is comparable to prevalence in individuals with chronic back pain. Therefore, it is recommended that those with moderate or severe pain symptoms be screened for psychiatric symptoms and illness-related disability to help ensure they are receiving holistic treatment. Screening measures may include use of the Generalized Anxiety Disorder scale (GAD-7) or the Short Health Anxiety Inventory to assess for symptoms of anxiety, or the Patient Health Questionnaire (PHQ-9) to assess for symptoms of depression. Self-screening measures are available on the internet (see the Resources for helpful links to self-screening measures) and can guide next steps as you talk with your medical provider about the role of anxiety or mood on your abdominal pain. Getting connected with a mental health provider can help you sort through the inner workings of the brain and how it deals with pain utilizing evidence-based psychological therapies.

Some mental health providers specialize in pain management and can serve as excellent members of your health-care team. Ask your medical provider for a referral to a health or pain psychologist. You can also use the directories in the Resources (pages 326–327).

Mind-Body and Brain-Gut Therapies

Cognitive behavioral therapy (CBT) is one of the most effective psychological therapies for those with abdominal pain. Treatment assists the client to identify maladaptive thoughts, perceptions, and behaviors. Training in relaxation skills is also a helpful component of treatment given the benefits of the body's relaxation response.

Sometimes, more **comprehensive pain rehabilitation** will involve physical therapy, occupational therapy, and CBT in an interdisciplinary outpatient setting. Most pain rehabilitation centers offer daily treatment for two to four weeks. The emphasis is on physical reconditioning and elimination of medications for pain (such as use of benzodiazepines). Complementary treatments such as acupuncture may also be suggested. Those who benefit from these types of programs do so because of a change in their behavior, beliefs, and physical status. While never a "quick fix," these programs empower people to change and effectively reduce pain.

Potential Future Therapy

A small study in IBS patients found that a **fecal microbial transplant** was able to improve symptoms of both depression and anxiety. While this therapy is not yet FDA approved for IBS, it may one day be available to help manage these often overlapping conditions.

ANXIETY

Anxiety is common in certain stressful situations, such as before taking a test, meeting a deadline, going to a job interview, or going on a first date. However, if anxiety begins to interfere with your ability to function due to feelings of excessive worry, dread, or fear, you may have an anxiety disorder.

The primary anxiety disorders that affect adults are generalized anxiety disorder (GAD), panic disorder (PD), social anxiety disorder (SAD), agoraphobia (fear of crowded places or of leaving the house), and specific phobias. Large reviews of scientific literature have found higher rates of anxiety in people who have IBS compared with those who do not have it. Given the potential for anxiety to worsen IBS symptoms and vice versa, it cannot be overlooked.

Anxiety: Additional Testing to Consider

If you believe you may be experiencing symptoms of anxiety, it may be helpful to use a self-reporting screening measures such as the GAD-7 (see the Resources for helpful links to self-screening measures). If your self-reported screening tool indicates anxiety, speak with a medical or mental health professional for additional assessment and to discuss treatment options.

Medications for Anxiety

In adults with GAD, selective serotonin reuptake inhibitors (SSRIs), serotonin-norepinephrine reuptake inhibitors (SNRIs), tricyclic antidepressants (TCAs), pregabalin, and benzodiazepines are commonly prescribed. You may work with a primary care physician to start medication for your anxiety. However, if you have not found relief and perhaps need a more comprehensive medication plan, we recommend consulting with a psychiatrist or psychiatric nurse practitioner.

Keep in mind that some anxiety medications can have digestive side effects. This can work in your favor in some instances and in others, not so much. You will need to talk to your prescribing provider. For example, SSRIs may cause or worsen diarrhea. TCAs may help alleviate diarrhea, but they may exacerbate constipation.

Diet Changes for Anxiety

A recent review evaluated the research on the diet-anxiety connection. It found that some key dietary patterns and food groups may help decrease anxiety, while others may worsen it. Unsurprisingly to us, a diet rich in certain substances—including fruits and veggies, specifically those that contain a wide range of polyphenols (we talk more about these important gut-friendly plant compounds in Chapter 10); healthy omega-3 fats (found in seeds, nuts, salmon); zinc, magnesium, and selenium (key minerals); and probiotics—helps in managing anxiety. So does eating breakfast! On the flip side, eating a diet rich in refined carbs (such as white flour and sugar) and high in fat but low in tryptophan (an amino acid found in poultry, milk, bananas, oats, peanuts) and in overall protein was associated with greater anxiety. Tryptophan is the precursor of serotonin, an important neurotransmitter that promotes emotional well-being and better attention and focus.

Psychological and Lifestyle Considerations for Anxiety

Psychological Therapies

Whether you start with medication or by seeing a therapist, know that anxiety is treatable. Lots of research shows that psychological therapies are effective for managing anxiety. Commonly applied therapies include **cognitive behavioral therapy (CBT)** and **acceptance and commitment therapy (ACT)**. As we have discussed throughout this book, CBT offers tools to improve your symptoms, decrease avoidance behaviors, and build your confidence in managing life's stressors. Treatment may also include aspects of exposure therapy, where you are gradually exposed to your anxiety triggers and provided with skills to manage the discomfort.

Additionally, a mental health provider can help you identify **lifestyle behaviors** that will support your long-term emotional and physical health. Walking, exercising, good sleep hygiene, spending time outside, socializing, and filling your body with nutritious food are all helpful when it comes to managing anxiety. If therapy alone does not provide adequate relief, talk with your doctor about the possibility of adding medication. To locate a mental health professional, see the Resources.

DEPRESSION

Just as we all experience periods of anxiety, symptoms of sadness or depression can be situational. In these instances—which last a short period of time—feeling the support of loved ones and refocusing your mind on other aspects of your life can often help lift the blues. However, persistent feelings of sadness, loss of interest, or hopelessness are signs of a mood disorder, also known as depression or major depressive disorder (MDD). Depression affects how you feel, think, and behave, which can lead to a variety of physical and emotional problems. It can impact your day-to-day functioning and may even make you feel as though you don't want to live anymore. Similar to anxiety, depression is more prevalent in people with IBS when compared to the general population; therefore, treatment of depression is an important step in the management of IBS.

Depression: Additional Testing to Consider

If you believe you are experiencing symptoms of depression, it may be helpful to use a self-reporting screening measure such as the PHQ-9 (see the Resources for links to self-screening measures). If your self-reported screening tool indicates symptoms of depression, speak with a medical or mental health professional. If you are experiencing thoughts of self-harm or suicide, please seek help immediately. Turn to page 326 for crisis intervention resources.

Medications for Depression

Currently, selective serotonin reuptake inhibitors (SSRIs, e.g., fluoxetine, sertraline, paroxetine, citalopram, and escitalopram) and serotonin-norepinephrine reuptake inhibitors (SNRIs, e.g., duloxetine, venlafaxine, and desvenlafaxine) are considered front-line pharmacological strategies for the medical treatment of depression. Other classes of medications are available too. We recommend working with your prescribing provider to outline a treatment plan specific to your needs.

Diet Changes for Depression

Yes, food can help your mood! Research has observed that adherence to a Mediterranean diet pattern—characterized by high consumption of fruits, vegetables, nuts, and legumes; moderate consumption of poultry, eggs, and dairy products; and only occasional consumption of red meat—is associated with a reduced risk of depression. As always, modify any type of eating plan to take into account your sensitivity to FODMAPs.

Psychological and Lifestyle Considerations

Psychological Therapies

Several types of psychological therapies can effectively address the distress associated with depression, including **cognitive behavioral therapy (CBT)**, **acceptance and commitment therapy (ACT)**, **dialectical behavioral therapy (DBT)**, and **interpersonal psychotherapy (ITP)**. It is important to talk with your mental health provider about their approach to the management of depression and how they will apply evidence-based interventions to help you learn to manage mood symptoms.

Several studies have shown that combining psychotherapy with antidepressant medications is associated with more favorable outcomes than psychotherapy or medication alone. It has been commonly suggested that medication may help initially stabilize symptoms of depression, whereas evidence-based psychotherapy provides longer-term intervention to manage mood and stabilize symptoms. The main takeaway is that depression is treatable, and life is very much worth living! Work with your medical team to find the strategies that work best for your depressive symptoms.

Patients often feel as though they have tried everything, and symptoms just aren't getting better. However, beginning to address your health by recognizing that food, lifestyle, mood, and more can all have an impact may open a door to evidence-based strategies that you hadn't considered before. Observe your symptoms, reflect on what you have tried, think about where you want to go next, and collaboratively work with your medical providers on your plan of action. Knowledge is power, and you've got the science-backed wisdom (and confidence) to start feeling better!

CHAPTER 10

IBS MIMICKERS, OR WHEN IBS OVERLAPS WITH OTHER CONDITIONS

IBS symptoms tend to be chronic in nature and exacerbated by stress. But it's not uncommon to wonder, as you sit on the toilet for the umpteenth time, if anything else could be going on. Indeed, there are other sneaky GI conditions that have symptoms similar to IBS and are often excluded in an IBS workup. They may be overlooked due to a lack of the appropriate testing at the medical center where you are being treated, or because the condition is in its earliest stages. The latter situation may occur with celiac disease (CD) or inflammatory bowel disease (IBD). A person with IBS symptoms may have a genetic propensity toward CD and IBD—the disease is brewing but the diagnosis is not yet fully evident.

It's also important to note that IBS may co-occur with other conditions. In other words, you may have IBS *and* something else. For instance, IBS-type symptoms occur in about 38 percent of CD patients, based on one scientific review. Likewise, IBS-like symptoms occur frequently in IBD patients, affecting about up to 40 percent.

Have you had a tendency to experience loose stools and urgent diarrhea since childhood? It could be the genetic condition associated with sucrase-isomaltase deficiency, a lack of an enzyme that digests sucrose. Did your symptoms start after you returned from a camping trip? It could be postinfectious IBS after a foodborne illness or perhaps a parasitic infection. Or maybe you recently had a baby? Dyssynergic defecation (DD) occurs when the muscles and nerves fail to work in a coordinated pattern, leading to challenges eliminating stool. This condition may present after childbirth because the muscles can be affected during delivery. With DD, it's like it's "opposite day": the gut muscles and nerves actually work *against* the natural process to eliminate stool, tightening and not relaxing.

In this chapter, we'll delve into common conditions that mimic or co-occur with IBS, including descriptions, common symptoms, how they are diagnosed, and their potential treatments.

CELIAC DISEASE

What it is: Celiac disease is a multisystem immune-mediated disorder resulting in damage to the small intestine when gluten is eaten. It occurs in genetically susceptible individuals. Gluten is a storage protein in wheat, rye, and barley. In people with CD, it drives gut inflammation and flattening of the absorptive areas (called villi) in the gut, leading to poor absorption of nutrients and GI symptoms.

Celiac disease is relatively uncommon, at least compared to IBS, occurring in about 1 percent of the North American population, although its prevalence is increasing. It affects more women than men.

Common symptoms: Diarrhea, bloating, constipation, and gastroesophageal reflux disease can occur in CD, but some people with the condition do not have any symptoms. Fatigue is common, possibly due to poor absorption of iron, vitamin B12, and zinc, nutrients that fuel the body's energy. Although CD primarily affects the gut, it is a complex disease that often presents with symptoms outside the GI system, including chronic fatigue, anemia, osteoporosis, ulcers in the mouth, elevated liver enzymes, joint pain, infertility, peripheral neuropathy, and even epilepsy.

How it's diagnosed: The diagnosis of CD is typically made by combining clinical symptoms, CD serology (blood) tests, and small intestinal biopsies—all while the patient is consuming a gluten-containing diet. Small intestinal biopsy remains the diagnostic gold standard for this condition.

It's important to note that consuming gluten is essential for the blood tests and small intestinal biopsies to be accurate in diagnosing celiac. If a celiac test is completed without adequate gluten intake, or perhaps if the testing does not provide clear results, genetic testing may provide some insights for ruling out CD. These genetic tests (HLA-DQ2 and HLA-DQ8) are useful because a negative test is highly predictive of a negative diagnosis. (It is less helpful if an individual tests positive for genetic markers for CD, as these markers occur in 25–35 percent of the general population, whereas only about 3 percent of those with positive gene tests will go on to develop CD.)

Treatment: Standard treatment is a strict, lifelong gluten-free diet, ideally reviewed in detail with the guidance of a GI expert dietitian. Given the importance of dietary adherence and because of other CD-related challenges, working with a GI psychologist as part of a treatment team can help with processing and gaining acceptance of living life with a chronic GI disease, managing stress, developing coping skills, improving emotional well-being, and overall quality of life.

INFLAMMATORY BOWEL DISEASE (CROHN'S DISEASE, ULCERATIVE COLITIS, MICROSCOPIC COLITIS)

What it is: Inflammatory bowel disease is a group of disorders involving chronic inflammation in the intestines. IBD includes Crohn's disease (which can present with inflammation in any part of the gastrointestinal tract, from mouth to anus), ulcerative colitis (in which the inflammation is limited to the colon), and microscopic colitis (in which inflammation is observed using a microscope). Microscopic colitis occurs more commonly in older patients and has two different subtypes, lymphocytic colitis and collagenous colitis. The prevalence of IBD is increasing globally and occurs in about 1.3 percent of Americans.

Common symptoms: Both Crohn's disease and ulcerative colitis typically present with abdominal pain and diarrhea. Rectal bleeding can also occur in both conditions but is more common in ulcerative colitis. Of those with IBD, 25 to 40 percent will experience complications that involve the skin, joints, eyes, kidneys, or liver.

How it's diagnosed: No single test is available to confirm the diagnosis of IBD. The gastroenterologist will start with blood and stool tests to look for inflammation markers. Blood tests include C-reactive protein (a CRP of ≤0.5 mg/dl makes a diagnosis of IBD less likely) and erythrocyte sedimentation rate (ESR). Stool tests include fecal calprotectin (<40 µg/g makes a diagnosis of IBD less likely) and lactoferrin. A colonoscopy (a small scope and camera inserted in the rectum to look at the colon) or an endoscopy (a small scope and camera inserted through the mouth into the esophagus, stomach, and small bowel) will be performed, and biopsies taken, to provide further information to help your clinician make the proper diagnosis.

Treatment: IBD is generally treated with a combination of medications (to suppress inflammation and lessen symptoms) and diet (to help manage symptoms while nourishing the body). In some cases, a formula-based diet can help get the inflammation under control. When scarring has occurred in the intestine, the patient might modify the types of dietary fiber they consume for better tolerance—for example, switching to more soluble fibers, or changing the consistency of fiber by blending or cooking foods. While diet is of great interest to patients and researchers alike in the treatment of IBD, we do not have solid ground for recommending a specific long-term diet therapy as a preventative or cure for IBD. Tailored diet therapy should involve a GI expert RD when possible. Mood and anxiety disorders are common in IBD, and the condition can have a profound impact on one's quality of life, so we recommend that a GI psychologist be part of the treatment team. Emotional health is just as important as physical health.

GI PARASITIC INFECTIONS

What it is: Parasites are organisms that live off other organisms to survive. Some parasitic infections do not result in GI distress, while others—notably infection caused by the microorganism giardia—may cause persistent IBS for years, even after effective treatment. One study revealed that 80.5 percent of individuals infected by giardia via contaminated water developed IBS symptoms. Once a person or animal has been infected with giardia, the parasite lives in the intestines and is passed in stool. Individuals should be tested for this condition if they are at greater risk, such as after travel in a developing country, following close contact with someone with giardiasis, after drinking unsafe water that hasn't been filtered, after camping (specifically swallowing water while swimming), and even after potential exposure in a childcare setting. Each year in the United States, it is estimated that giardia causes more than 1.1 million illnesses.

Common symptoms: Bloating, diarrhea, and abdominal pain.

How it's diagnosed: Stool tests: fecal immunoassays or polymerase chain reaction tests. Because giardia can be difficult to detect, at least three stool specimens, collected on different days, should be examined to confirm its presence.

Treatment: Antibiotics and antiparasitic medications.

BILE ACID DIARRHEA

What it is: Bile acid diarrhea (BAD) is a common cause of chronic diarrhea, affecting about 1 percent of the general population and up to 50 percent of those with IBS-D. BAD is also common in ileal Crohn's disease or after an ileal resection. ("Ileal" means having to do with the ileum, which is the third section of the small intestine.) It is characterized by excess bile acids in the colon, resulting in increased colonic motility and fluid secretion. Bile acids are made in the liver, stored in the gallbladder, and released into the intestine to help with the digestion and absorption of fat. Bile acid diarrhea can result due to overproduction of bile acids, malabsorption of bile acids due to intestinal resection, or small intestinal bacterial overgrowth (the surplus bacteria render the bile acids inactive).

Common symptoms: Urgent diarrhea is the primary symptom of BAD. Poorly absorbed bile acids pull water into the gut and accelerate colonic movement, leading to urgency. Symptoms of bile acid malabsorption differ from IBS in that the urgency to use the bathroom can occur at night (IBS symptoms don't usually happen at night).

How it's diagnosed: Many clinical practices administer a trial treatment of bile acid binders (also known as bile acid sequestrants). If they work, the diagnosis of bile acid diarrhea is confirmed. Clinical tests for the condition include 75-selenium homocholic acid taurine (SeHCAT), serum C4, fibroblast growth factor 19 (FGF-19), and measurement of fecal bile acids excretion.

Treatment: Bile acid binders (e.g., cholestyramine and colestipol) are commonly used to treat this condition.

SUCRASE-ISOMALTASE DEFICIENCY

What it is: Sucrase-isomaltase deficiency (SID) occurs when there is an absence of (or decline in) the enzymes responsible for digesting sucrose (found in table sugar, pastries, sweets, and naturally in some fruits and vegetables) and certain starches (found in rice, potatoes, bread, pasta). How the condition manifests depends on the person's genes. In congenital sucrase-isomaltase deficiency (CSID), a child inherits genes from both parents that affect the production of the enzyme. CSID is often diagnosed during childhood. People with IBS appear to have a higher incidence of alterations in their genes for SID. However, a person may inherit the gene from only one parent and experience less severe symptoms. It is estimated that as many as one in ten people diagnosed with IBS-D may have SID.

Common symptoms: Diarrhea, abdominal pain, distention, and cramps upon ingestion of sugar. When sucrase-isomaltase is absent or deficient, unabsorbed carbohydrates enter the latter part of the small intestine and colon, where they ferment, leading to excessive production of acids and gases.

How it's diagnosed: The gold standard test for this condition is a biopsy of the duodenum (first part of the small intestine) to test for the levels of disaccharidase digestive enzymes.

Treatment: An enzyme supplement can be prescribed, but it only covers sucrose digestion. For patients with starch intolerance, a registered dietitian can provide guidance on modifying starchy foods.

SMALL INTESTINAL BACTERIAL OVERGROWTH

What it is: The latest American College of Gastroenterology clinical guidelines for small intestinal bacterial overgrowth (SIBO) define the condition as the presence of excessive numbers of bacteria in the small bowel, causing gastrointestinal symptoms. SIBO is described in detail in Chapter 8.

How it's diagnosed: A breath test for lactulose or glucose is the most common diagnostic tool. Less typically, a culture of the small bowel via an endoscope may be taken to assess for abnormal numbers of microorganisms.

Common symptoms: Bloating is the most common symptom of SIBO, but other IBS symptoms are often present, such as abdominal pain and alterations in bowel habit. The excess gas and bloating are caused by unhealthy fermentation of nutrients by the surplus bacteria in the small intestine.

Treatment: Antibiotic therapies may be used. Ideally, the underlying cause is identified, such as untreated celiac disease, severe constipation, or untreated thyroid condition. To achieve prolonged remission, it's important to treat the underlying cause when possible. Modifying intake of fermentable foods may help reduce clinical symptoms, but this has not been formally studied in the research setting.

EXOCRINE PANCREATIC INSUFFICIENCY

What it is: The pancreas normally produces enzymes that help the body digest foods. Exocrine pancreatic insufficiency (EPI) occurs when the pancreas fails to produce enough of these enzymes, resulting in maldigestion of foods and food intolerance. One study found that EPI is present in 5 percent of patients who fulfill the Rome Foundation's criteria for IBS-D.

Common symptoms: Abdominal pain, gas, bloating, constipation, diarrhea, and fatty stools (stools that are lighter in color, float, and are more odorous). Dyspepsia, a symptom of indigestion involving pain or a feeling of discomfort in the upper abdomen, is strongly associated with EPI.

How it's diagnosed: Common tests for EPI include the fecal elastase test (FE-1) to check stool for the presence of the enzyme elastase, which helps to digest protein, fat, and carbohydrates. Little or no elastase can indicate EPI. A fecal fat test might be conducted to measure the amount of fat in stool. A high volume of fat may be a sign of EPI.

Treatment: EPI is treated with pancreatic enzyme replacement therapy, also known as PERT.

DYSSYNERGIC DEFECATION

What it is: Dyssynergic defecation (DD) occurs when there is an inability to coordinate the abdominal and pelvic floor muscles to evacuate stool. This is often described as a paradoxical contraction because it is the opposite of what helps eliminate stool from the rectum. DD occurs in about 50 percent of those who experience constipation. Excessive straining to expel hard stools may over time lead to dyssynergic defecation.

How it's diagnosed: The primary tests for DD include anorectal manometry and the balloon expulsion test. A clinical history and careful rectal examination can be a preliminary gauge to raise suspicion of the disorder.

Common symptoms: Symptoms include incomplete evacuation, straining, and prolonged toileting. A high stool burden (a colon full of stool) related to pelvic floor dysfunction and DD can trigger bloating, cramping, and incomplete emptying, common symptoms in individuals with IBS.

Treatment: Pelvic floor physical therapy and biofeedback; see the Resources for help finding a pelvic floor physical therapist.

It is essential to have trust in your health-care team to actively listen to you, help guide you to find the best treatments, and potentially assess you for IBS mimickers. You are the expert about your body, but the medical experts will work with you to determine a plan for diagnosis and treatment that is evidence-based and applies the gold standard in care. When you are comfortable with your medical team, the process of determining which health conditions are playing a part in your clinical presentation will be smoother.

No one knows your body better than you! Listen to it, remember that your gut is your second brain, and have the confidence to advocate for yourself if you feel something has been missed or you haven't received a proper explanation for your symptoms. As they say, teamwork makes the dream work, and for addressing your GI symptoms, that team may include more people than simply you and your physician. With the correct team in place, all of you can work effectively together to determine appropriate next steps on your healing journey.

THE LAST WORDS

"I finally understand this diagnosis and recognize that there are ways I can improve and get my life back. I feel hopeful for the first time in a long time."

—Jen

"I can't believe it took me this long to receive life-changing tips and tricks for two things I have been doing my entire life: eating and going to the bathroom. I can enjoy both now."

—Michael

If you are a runner, you may have a favorite pair of shoes that you slide on before you hit the road for a quick jaunt. For a longer run, you may take along a few more essentials, such as your earbuds, lip balm, a water bottle, and a watch. In the same way, as you work to incorporate stress management, relaxation, diet changes, and self-care into your life, you may find yourself bringing along several favorite strategies.

We encourage you to keep a list of the IBS management strategies that you find most helpful and enjoyable. If you haven't already done so, write them down in the back of this book on the Mind Your Gut My Essentials for Health List (page 317). Include the page number where you found the strategy so you can return to it until you've achieved mastery. As you are probably finding with all the Mind Your Gut tools, improvements in IBS are possible. They may already be happening for you! Armed with a list of essentials, if you have a return of tummy troubles, need a mindset tune-up, or want a refresher on a delicious recipe, you can easily return to the tools that help you mind that gut.

IBS is a chronic and unpredictable condition. However, consistent use of the techniques you are learning can result in symptoms that are less frequent, less severe, and less anxiety-provoking. The tools in your toolbox will never go away—and neither will your ability to manage IBS (or life's other stressors). You are empowered to deal with symptoms if they come on. That is the true goal! We want you to feel the invigorating effects of these life changes on your overall health and well-being. Think of the strategies for managing nutrition and stress as a lifestyle you are adopting for the long run.

Thank you for allowing us to be members on your team. It's been a pleasure to be a part of your healing journey, and we wish you the very best.

APPENDIX I

GUT-LOVING RECIPES

Not everyone loves to cook, we get it. So we kept the recipes in this section quick and easy to make, gut-friendly, and low-FODMAP. Consider trying one or two recipes a week to expand your diet and enjoy some new food combos. Remember to add the ingredients from the recipes you intend to try to your weekly grocery list to be sure you have what you need to whip up some deliciousness.

The recipes in this section feature nutrients that promote gut health while being low in FODMAPs to keep your gut soothed and calm. Recipes are noted with special icons to identify when they fit other special diet considerations:

V = vegan
VN = vegetarian (may include dairy and eggs)
GF = gluten-free
DF = dairy-free

BREAKFAST IDEAS

Low-FODMAP Seedy Granola

The seeds in the granola offer up additional magnesium, polyphenols, healthy fats, and fiber to promote a healthy gut microbiome. Magnesium is an important mineral that helps support nerves, muscles, and proper gut function (and that most of us fall short on).

V, VN, GF, DF

Makes about 8 servings | Serving size: 1/2 cup

2 cups old-fashioned oats (use certified GF oats if following a GF diet)

1 cup millet (uncooked)

1 cup pepitas (hulled pumpkin seeds)

¼ cup sunflower seeds

⅓ cup maple syrup

½ cup melted coconut oil

1 teaspoon vanilla extract

¼ cup shredded unsweetened coconut

1. Preheat the oven to 300°F.

2. Line a rimmed baking sheet with parchment paper.

3. In a medium bowl, stir all ingredients together until well combined. Spread the mixture in an even layer on the baking sheet.

4. Bake for 45 minutes, stirring midway through. Remove from the oven and allow to cool to room temperature.

5. Place cooled granola in an airtight container, and use within seven days.

Banana Pumpkin Blender Muffins

These flavorful, whole-grain, oat-based muffins provide about 5 grams of gut-loving fiber per muffin. The amount of ripe banana included per serving makes this a low-FODMAP treat.

VN, GF, DF

Makes 7 large (Texas-size muffin pan) or 9 regular (standard muffin pan) muffins | Serving size: 1 muffin (large or standard)

1 cup pumpkin puree

1 medium-sized ripe banana

3 tablespoons water

2 large eggs

2 cups old-fashioned oats (use certified GF oats if following a GF diet)

¼ cup extra virgin olive oil

3 tablespoons maple syrup

1 teaspoon cinnamon

¼ teaspoon ground cloves

¼ teaspoon allspice

1 teaspoon baking soda

Toppings (optional): chia seeds, chopped walnuts or pecans, sunflower seeds, dark chocolate chips (use DF chocolate if following a DF diet)

1. Preheat the oven to 350°F. Lightly oil a muffin tin and set aside, or place a paper liner in each cup.

2. Place all ingredients except toppings in a large blender. Pulse the blender, stopping to stir as needed, until the mixture is well blended and creamy.

3. Pour the batter into the prepared muffin pan, filling each cup about three-quarters full. (A standard muffin pan will require about ¼ cup of batter per muffin, and a Texas-size muffin pan will require about ⅓ cup of batter per muffin.) Sprinkle about 1 tablespoon of nuts, seeds, chocolate chips, or a combo on the top of each muffin.

4. Bake for 25–35 minutes, or until a toothpick inserted in the center of a muffin comes out with just a few damp crumbs clinging to it. Baking time will vary depending on muffin size.

Green Goddess Smoothie

The green goodness in this flavorful smoothie is from a low-FODMAP veggie powerhouse: spinach.

V, VN, GF, DF

Serves 1

1 frozen banana (firm/ unripe)

1 tablespoon almond butter

1 cup spinach

1 tablespoon unsalted sunflower seeds

½ cup almond milk

5 baby carrots

1 tablespoon grated fresh ginger

2 teaspoons maple syrup

Blend ingredients in a high-speed blender until creamy. Add water or ice to reach desired consistency. (If you don't have a high-speed blender, finely chop the banana and carrots first.)

Clean-Sweep Take-2 Smoothie

The goal of this bowel-busting smoothie is to help keep you regular. Each serving contains two entire kiwifruits, which have been shown in multiple studies to fend off constipation.

V, VN, GF, DF

Serves 1

2 green kiwifruits, peeled (fresh or chopped frozen)

1 cup kale leaves, stems removed (or use baby kale)

⅛ avocado

½ cup diced frozen pineapple

1 tablespoon hemp seeds

2 teaspoons chia seeds

Water/ice to blend to desired consistency

Blend all ingredients in a blender until creamy and smooth, adding ice and water as needed.

From-the-Garden Egg Cups

Eating a variety of vegetables helps keep your gut microbiota diverse and healthy. This breakfast dish offers a delicious way to start your day.

VN, GF
Serves 6

1 tablespoon extra-virgin olive oil

1 cup diced broccoli florets

½ cup diced summer squash

1 cup fresh baby spinach leaves

5 large eggs

¼ cup lactose-free milk

(rice milk or other low-FODMAP unsweetened milk can be substituted)

½ cup grated cheddar or Swiss cheese

¼ teaspoon dried basil

¼ teaspoon dried oregano

Salt and pepper

1. Preheat the oven to 350°F. Lightly oil six cups of a muffin tin and set aside.

2. In a large skillet over medium heat, combine the olive oil, broccoli, squash, and spinach. Sauté the vegetables until fork-tender, about 5 minutes. Drain any excess liquid from the mixture.

3. In a medium bowl, combine the eggs, milk, cheese, basil, oregano, and a pinch each of salt and pepper. Whisk ingredients together until blended.

4. Divide the veggie mixture evenly among the six greased muffin cups. Top with the egg-and-cheese mixture, filling each cup about three-quarters full.

5. Bake for 20–30 minutes or until the eggs are set and cooked through.

6. Let cool for about 10 minutes. Remove the egg cups from the tin, running a butter knife around the edge of each egg cup to loosen it.

Morning Oat Bowl

We love oats! They tend to be gentler on the gut than most other grains, and they offer up beta-glucan, a favorite food source for our health-promoting gut microbes. Tip: If using steel-cut oats, which are a bit more durable than old-fashioned rolled oats, make several servings when meal prepping, and store the extra cooked oats in an airtight container in the refrigerator. The oats can be used throughout the week. Simply reheat them in the microwave, and add your topping of choice.

Serves 1

Cook oats according to package directions. Top 1 cup of cooked oats with one of the following combos:

Pomegranate and seeds bowl

¼ cup pomegranate arils

1 tablespoon pumpkin seeds

2 teaspoons chia seeds

Fruit and nut butter bowl

1 cup blueberries

1 tablespoon all-natural peanut butter

2 teaspoons sunflower seeds

Carrot cake bowl

¾ cup grated carrots

1 tablespoon unsweetened shredded coconut

1 tablespoon chopped pecans

Sprinkle of cinnamon

Banana Pancakes

These yummy, kid-approved pancakes are simple to make in the blender. Plus they contain whole-grain, gut-friendly oats.

VN, GF, DF

Serves 3–4

2 medium unripe bananas

2 large eggs

3 tablespoons maple syrup

1½ cups old-fashioned rolled oats (use certified GF oats if following a GF diet)

½ teaspoon baking powder

½ teaspoon cinnamon

2 tablespoons extra-virgin olive oil

1. Place all ingredients in a blender. Pulse until the mixture reaches batter consistency. Add water if necessary to thin it a bit.

2. Heat a large, lightly oiled skillet or griddle over medium heat.

3. Pour the batter onto the griddle in rounds, measuring about ⅓ cup for each pancake. Flip the pancakes when lightly browned on the sides. Remove from heat when cooked through and golden brown. Repeat with remaining batter.

LUNCH AND DINNER IDEAS

Zesty Lentil Soup

Canned lentils contain fewer FODMAPs than the dried-and-boiled versions. You'll love the ease of preparing this recipe—dinner will be served in minutes!

V, VN, GF, DF

Serves 3

1 tablespoon shallot-infused or plain extra-virgin olive oil

1 cup diced carrots

½ cup diced zucchini

1 cup canned diced tomatoes (we love fire-roasted tomatoes), liquid included

1 cup canned lentils, drained and rinsed (about a 15-ounce can)

2 cups low-FODMAP chicken or vegetable broth (use vegetable broth if following a vegan or vegetarian diet and GF broth if following a GF diet)

½ teaspoon cumin

Hot sauce, optional (we like Texas Pete's)

1. In a medium stockpot, heat the olive oil over medium-high heat until shimmering. Add the diced carrots and zucchini, and cook, stirring occasionally, until the vegetables are fork-tender, about 10 minutes. (The zucchini will cook faster than the carrots.) Stir in the tomatoes, lentils, broth, and cumin. Simmer for about 15 minutes, or until some of the liquid has evaporated and the soup has a hearty appearance.

2. Serve with a splash of hot sauce, if desired.

Carrot Ginger Soup

Kate's go-to recipe for IBS-flare management, this gentle soup is a great gut soother. You'll love its flavor and creaminess. Make a batch and freeze some to have on hand when you need a little gut love.

GF, DF

Serves 6

8 cups chopped carrots (about 16 medium carrots)

5 cups reduced-sodium, reduced-fat, low-FODMAP chicken broth (use GF broth if following a GF diet)

1 tablespoon minced ginger, fresh or jarred

Salt and pepper to taste

1. Combine carrots, broth, and ginger in a large stockpot over high heat. Bring to a boil. Reduce heat to medium, and simmer until the carrots are fork-tender, about 20 minutes. Add salt and pepper. Remove soup from the heat, and let it cool for about 20 minutes.

2. Once the soup is cooled, pour enough into a blender to fill it about two-thirds. (Don't attempt to blend hot liquid!) Blend until creamy, and pour the blended soup into a fresh stockpot to rewarm it. Blend the remainder of the soup in batches.

Farmers' Market Pasta

This veggie-loaded pasta salad is a family fave! It checks all the gut-love boxes: high in prebiotic fiber, includes a diversity of veggies, adds just enough prebiotic-rich legumes, and contains a nice dose of healthy fats.

V, VN, GF, DF

Serves 4

6 ounces suitable GF pasta or low-FODMAP GF pasta

1 green bell pepper, deseeded and sliced into strips

2 carrots, peeled and sliced into thin rounds

10 cherry tomatoes, sliced in half

1 cup canned chickpeas, drained and rinsed

½ cup pitted kalamata olives

2 tablespoons chopped fresh basil

Lemon dressing

Juice of 1 lemon (about 2 tablespoons)

¼ cup garlic-infused or plain extra-virgin olive oil

Salt and pepper to taste

1. Prepare the pasta according to package directions. Drain and rinse, and place in a medium bowl. Add the bell pepper, carrots, tomatoes, chickpeas, olives, and basil, stirring to combine.

2. In a small bowl, whisk together the dressing ingredients. While the pasta is still warm, pour the dressing over the pasta mixture, and lightly toss to combine.

Garden Veggie Burger

You won't miss the beef in this flavorful, prebiotic-rich burger. For a vegan variation, use a flax substitute for the egg. Mix 1 tablespoon flaxseed meal with 2 1/2 tablespoons water; let sit for 5 minutes to thicken.

V (option), VN, GF, DF

Serves 4

1 cup canned lentils, drained and rinsed

1 cup cooked quinoa

½ cup old-fashioned oats (use certified GF oats if following a GF diet)

1 large carrot, grated

¼ red bell pepper, diced (this amount is low enough in FODMAPs)

1 egg, lightly whisked (see above for a vegan variation)

Extra-virgin olive oil

1 teaspoon suitable taco seasoning (see Resources section; use GF if following a GF diet)

1. Place the lentils, quinoa, and oats in a blender, and pulse just enough to blend. You want some texture, but blending a little bit will help the burgers stick together. Spoon the mixture into a medium mixing bowl. Fold in the carrot and red pepper. Add the egg (or the flax substitute), and stir to combine.

2. Form 4 burger patties with your hands. Place them on a parchment-lined tray, cover with plastic wrap, and refrigerate long enough for the mixture to set, about 1 hour.

3. Lightly oil a medium skillet over medium heat, and slide the burgers into the skillet. Cook for 3–5 minutes, flip, and cook the other side until the patties are heated through and a light crust has formed on each side.

Chicken Quinoa Meatballs with Brown Rice Noodles and Carrots

Quinoa adds a nice dose of fiber and protein to these delicious, gut-friendly meatballs.

GF, DF

Serves 4

Meatballs

Extra-virgin olive oil

1 pound ground chicken breast

2 cups cooked quinoa, drained of any extra liquid

1 egg yolk

2 tablespoons soy sauce (use GF if following a GF diet; we like reduced-sodium San-J Tamari)

1 tablespoon sesame oil

1 teaspoon ground ginger (or 3–4 tablespoons grated fresh ginger)

1 tablespoon hot sauce (choose one without onion or garlic; our favorite is Texas Pete's)

Soy Sesame Drizzle

¼ cup soy sauce (use GF if following a GF diet)

1 tablespoon rice vinegar

½ teaspoon ground ginger or 2 tablespoons grated fresh ginger

1 tablespoon light brown sugar

1 teaspoon sesame oil

1 teaspoon cornstarch whisked into ¼ cup water

Garnish

2 cups cooked brown rice noodles, warmed

2 cups steamed or sautéed baby carrots

1 tablespoon toasted sesame seeds

1–2 tablespoons sliced scallions (green part only)

¼ cup chopped cilantro leaves, optional

1. Preheat the oven to 350°F. Lightly oil a large baking sheet.

2. In a medium bowl, mix together the ground chicken, quinoa, egg yolk, soy sauce, sesame oil, ginger, and hot sauce until well combined. Form the mixture into 50 small meatballs. Arrange the meatballs close to one another on a baking sheet. Bake for 18–20 minutes or until cooked through.

3. While the meatballs are cooking, make the Soy Sesame Drizzle. In a small saucepan over medium-low heat, stir together the soy sauce, rice vinegar, ginger, brown sugar, and sesame oil. Once the mixture is warm, slowly add the cornstarch mixture, whisking constantly. Continue to cook, stirring occasionally, until the sauce thickens to a gravy-like consistency, about 5 minutes. Remove from heat.

4. Place the noodles and carrots on a platter. Top with the cooked meatballs. Lightly pour the Soy Sesame Drizzle over the meatballs. Sprinkle with sesame seeds, scallions, and cilantro leaves (if desired).

Shrimp Fried Rice
with Kimchi Topping

If you use precooked brown rice (often located in the freezer section of the grocery store) and frozen shrimp that has been peeled and deveined, this dish can whip up quickly. We include a small amount of kimchi, a type of fermented cabbage originally from Korea (staying within the low-FODMAP guidelines, of course). This adds flavor and a dose of fermented foods, which have been shown to increase the gut's microbial diversity. You can find kimchi in the refrigerated produce section of most large grocery stores and in Asian markets.

GF, DF

Serves 4

2 tablespoons sesame oil, divided

1 tablespoon garlic-infused or plain extra-virgin olive oil

About 16 extra-large shrimp, peeled and deveined (thawed if frozen)

1 cup broccoli florets, chopped into bite-size pieces

1 cup thinly sliced carrot rounds

2 large eggs

4 cups cooked brown rice, cooled

¼ cup soy sauce (use GF if following a GF diet)

½ cup kimchi

1 tablespoon toasted sesame seeds, optional

1. In a large skillet over medium heat, heat 1 tablespoon sesame oil and all the olive oil until shimmering. Add the shrimp and cook for 1–2 minutes, until pink and opaque. Remove shrimp to a plate.

2. Add the remaining 1 tablespoon sesame oil to the skillet along with the vegetables. Cook for about 3 minutes or until the vegetables are fork-tender.

3. Move the veggies to one side of the skillet. Crack the eggs into the empty part of the skillet, and scramble with a spatula until

cooked through, about 3 minutes. Add the cooked rice and the soy sauce, stirring to combine. Return the shrimp to the pan to heat through.

4.   Top with 2 tablespoons kimchi per serving. Serve with a sesame seed garnish, if desired.

Confetti Rice

Who doesn't like a sprinkle of confetti? The colorful veggies add a bit of fun and good nutrition to this tasty rice dish. If you wish, turn it into a complete meal by topping it with a protein: canned chickpeas, canned lentils, or grilled chicken breast or salmon.

V, VN, GF, DF
Serves 4

2 tablespoons garlic- or shallot-infused extra-virgin olive oil (or plain)

2 cups cooked brown rice

2 large carrots, finely chopped

1 cup finely chopped red cabbage

1 cup finely chopped broccoli florets

1 tablespoon soy sauce, optional (use GF if following a GF diet)

2 teaspoons fresh lemon juice

Salt and pepper to taste

Heat the olive oil in a large skillet over medium heat until shimmering. Add the cooked rice. Cook, stirring, until the rice is warmed through. Stir in the carrots, cabbage, and broccoli. Add 2 tablespoons water to the pan, and stir to combine. Cover the skillet and cook the vegetables until crisp-tender, 3–5 minutes, stirring midway through. Drizzle with soy sauce (if using) and lemon juice, and season with salt and pepper.

Crispy Almond Baked Chicken Tenders

These chicken tenders get a makeover: they're prepared with almond flour and delectably seasoned.

GF, DF

Serves 4

1 cup almond flour

1 teaspoon dried oregano

1 teaspoon dried basil

Salt and pepper to taste

1 large egg

1 pound skinless, boneless chicken breast, sliced into desired serving sizes (tenders or nuggets)

Oil spray, such as avocado or olive oil

1. Preheat the oven to 350°F. Line a rimmed baking sheet with parchment paper and set aside.

2. Stir together the almond flour, oregano, basil, salt, and pepper on a medium plate. Whisk the egg with 1 tablespoon water in a small bowl. Working a couple of pieces at a time, place the chicken in the egg mixture, then lightly dredge the pieces in the almond flour. Arrange the chicken on the baking sheet.

3. Bake for 10 minutes. Remove from the oven, and lightly spray the chicken with the oil spray. Using a spatula or tongs, flip the chicken pieces, and return them to the oven for 10 minutes or until cooked through (smaller pieces will take less time than larger pieces; adjust cooking time accordingly).

SNACKS AND TREATS

Low-FOD Lemony Hummus

Store-bought hummus is often laden with garlic (a common FODMAP trigger), but this hummus has all the delicious garlic flavor while fitting the criteria for the low-FODMAP elimination diet. Garlic-infused oil is the secret ingredient!

V, VN, GF, DF

Makes 4 servings

1 cup canned chickpeas, drained and rinsed

2 tablespoons freshly squeezed lemon juice

¼ cup tahini, well-stirred

1 teaspoon cumin

2 tablespoons garlic-infused extra-virgin olive oil

Salt to taste

Paprika for garnish

1. Place chickpeas, lemon juice, tahini, cumin, olive oil, and salt in a blender. Pulse to blend, adding 1–2 tablespoons water to thin to desired consistency.

2. Serve in a small bowl, topped with a sprinkle of paprika. Enjoy with baby carrots, sliced cucumber, bell pepper slices, or corn tortilla chips.

Small-Batch Almond Flour Dark Chocolate Chip Cookies

There is no wheat in these delish almond flour cookies, making them suitable for gluten-free and low-FODMAP dietary needs.

VN, GF

Makes 16 cookies | Serving size: 2 cookies

⅓ cup unsalted butter, at room temperature

⅓ cup light brown sugar

1 teaspoon vanilla

1 large egg

2 cups finely ground almond flour

½ teaspoon baking soda

⅓ cup dark chocolate morsels

¼ cup chopped walnuts

1. In a medium bowl, cream butter and sugar. Add vanilla and egg, mixing to blend.

2. Mix in almond flour and baking soda until creamy. Fold in chocolate morsels and walnuts.

3. Cover the bowl in plastic wrap and place in the refrigerator to set the dough, about 1 hour.

4. When the dough is set, preheat the oven to 350°F.

5. Line a rimmed baking sheet with parchment paper. Roll dough into small balls, and arrange them on the baking sheet about 2 inches apart.

6. Bake for 8–10 minutes, or until the cookies are slightly brown on the edges. Let cool and enjoy!

Almond Cranberry Energy Bites

Made with oats, these little bites are full of beta-glucan, providing fiber and prebiotics for gut health.

V, VN, GF, DF

Makes 18 bites | Serving size: 1 bite

1⅓ cups rolled oats (use certified GF oats if following a GF diet)

¼ cup sliced almonds

½ cup peanut butter

¼ cup maple syrup

¼ cup dried cranberries, roughly chopped

1 tablespoon chia seeds

½ teaspoon almond extract

1. Preheat the oven to 325°F.

2. Spread the oats and almonds evenly on a cookie sheet. Bake for 5–7 minutes or until lightly toasted, stirring midway through.

3. Place the oats and nuts in a medium mixing bowl. Add the remaining ingredients, and stir well to blend.

4. Cover a small tray with parchment paper. Roll the mixture into 18 bite-size balls, and arrange them on the tray. Refrigerate the bites until set, about 1 hour. Store in an airtight container in the refrigerator for up to a week.

Peanut Butter Dark Chocolate Chip Energy Bites

Nothing beats the combo of chocolate and peanut butter—and these bites afford gut-loving benefits! They include prebiotics from the oats, polyphenols from the dark chocolate, and of course fiber and healthy fats from the peanut butter.

V, VN, GF, DF

Makes 18 balls | Serving size: 2 balls

1½ cups rolled oats (use certified GF oats if following a GF diet)

⅓ cup shredded unsweetened coconut

½ cup creamy natural peanut butter

¼ cup maple syrup

2 tablespoons chia seeds

1 tablespoon ground flaxseed

¼ cup dark chocolate chips, roughly chopped (use DF chips if following a DF or vegan diet)

1. In a medium bowl, stir together the oats, coconut, peanut butter, maple syrup, chia seeds, and flaxseed until well blended. Fold in the chocolate chips.

2. Roll into about 18 balls, placing them on a tray lined with parchment paper. Refrigerate to set, about 1 hour. Store in an airtight container in the refrigerator for up to a week.

Raw Brownie Rounds

These little nuggets of gut love taste so decadent. They are made with fiber-rich walnuts and polyphenol-rich cocoa—food sources for those good gut microbes! Note: This recipe requires a strong blender or medium-sized food processor to create the desired thick, creamy consistency of the batter.

V, VN, GF, DF
Makes 10 brownie bites | Serving size: 1 bite

1 cup walnut halves

½ cup raisins

¼ cup cocoa powder (e.g., Hershey's Special Dark cocoa)

1 teaspoon vanilla extract

1 tablespoon maple syrup

Optional garnishes: hemp seeds, chia seeds, shredded coconut, mini semisweet chocolate chips (use DF chocolate chips if following a DF or vegan diet)

1. Place walnuts, raisins, cocoa powder, vanilla, and maple syrup in a strong blender or food processor fit with the metal blade. Pulse to blend, slowly adding about 2 teaspoons water to thin the batter. Note: The batter should be thicker than traditional brownie batter—it needs to stay in the shape of a ball.

2. Roll the mixture into about 10 evenly sized balls. Roll each ball in one of the garnish options, if desired. Store in an airtight container in the refrigerator for up to a week.

Oatmeal Cookie Smoothie

All the flavors of an oatmeal cookie packaged up in a smoothie rich with pre-biotic fibers and fermented ingredients for your long-term gut health.

VN, GF

Serves 1

½ cup plain or vanilla lactose-free kefir (without inulin or chicory root additives)

1 frozen banana (just ripe)

⅓ cup rolled oats (use certified GF oats if following a GF diet)

1 tablespoon raisins

½ teaspoon cinnamon

Place all ingredients in a blender. Blend the mixture until creamy, adding water or ice to reach desired consistency.

Power Sport Smoothie

We use protein-rich (lactose-free) Greek yogurt in this smoothie concoction. It was created for the person living an active lifestyle to simultaneously fuel muscles and gut microbiome.

VN, GF

Serves 1

1 unripe banana, frozen

1 cup lactose-free plain Greek yogurt

2 tablespoons peanut butter

1 cup frozen blueberries

1–2 teaspoons maple syrup, to taste (optional)

Place all ingredients in a blender. Blend the mixture until creamy, adding water or ice to reach desired consistency.

SALAD DRESSINGS

Maple Dijon Dressing

A popular homemade dressing that contains only natural ingredients: no manufactured additives or thickeners. And zero onion or garlic to potentially wreak havoc on your gut symptoms.

V, VN, GF, DF

Serves 2

3 tablespoons fresh-squeezed lemon juice

¼ cup extra-virgin olive oil

1 tablespoon maple syrup

2 teaspoons Dijon mustard (without onion or garlic)

Salt and pepper to taste

Whisk all ingredients together in a small bowl. Serve immediately.

Asian Sesame Dressing

Flavorful for salads, as a marinade, or over rice noodles. You'll love this dressing that has no added sugar but does have a little kick!

V, VN, GF, DF

Serves 2

¼ cup toasted sesame oil

1 tablespoon garlic-infused (or plain) extra-virgin olive oil

2 tablespoons rice vinegar

2 tablespoons soy sauce (use GF if following a GF diet)

1 teaspoon crushed red pepper (optional)

Whisk all ingredients together in a small bowl. Serve immediately.

APPENDIX II

COLONOSCOPY-COPING PREP KIT

Undergoing a colonoscopy is the most effective way to prevent colon cancer and to screen for other GI diseases, such as colitis, inflammatory bowel disease, or diverticulosis. Mainly, the gastroenterologist is looking for precancerous or cancerous polyps in the colon that they will remove and test. People with health-specific anxiety or a history of trauma sometimes avoid medical procedures like colonoscopy. (In fact, fear of a cancer diagnosis has been shown in research to contribute to high levels of anxiety in 22–55 percent of people undergoing a colonoscopy.) But given that this procedure can be lifesaving, we urge you to keep your appointment. And we firmly believe that the strategies outlined here will help you emotionally and physically with the colon prep.

1) Talk with your doctor about what makes you nervous: the prep, the sedation, getting an IV, complications with the procedure, the sensitive nature of the procedure, or embarrassment during the procedure. Having an open conversation with your doctor can help the medical team provide you with more information to assist in

calming your concerns. Ask for educational pamphlets and informational videos to gain a better understanding of the colonoscopy experience.

Here is an example of a short, informative video: "Preparing for Your GI Procedure" (from University of Michigan Health), www.uofmhealth.org/conditions-treatments/digestive-and-liver -health/preparing-your-gi-procedure.

2) If you have a phobia of needles or injections, when you show up for your colonoscopy, let the medical providers know. You are not alone. They can assist in making you comfortable. They may describe what to expect in a bit more detail, help distract you with some humorous dialogue, or allow you to use relaxation skills while they prep you for the procedure.

3) Activate your relaxation response. As you wait for the procedure, you can use diaphragmatic breathing or another form of relaxed breathing. Practice your relaxation strategies regularly so you feel comfortable implementing them on the day of your procedure.

4) Make a playlist of your favorite music. Listening to your tunes of choice while waiting for the procedure can ease worry.

5) Focus on the positives. When you avoid things that your doctor wants you to do, it often adds to stress. By following through on this important medical procedure, you are taking steps to proactively manage your health. Whatever the results of the colonoscopy, you will use that information to focus on the next steps of treatment.

Colonoscopy Prep:
Low-FODMAP Clear-Liquid Inspirations

Reminder: Always check ingredient labels as manufacturers can change ingredients at any time.

- Jell-O brand boxed lemon gelatin (sweetened with sugar; make it yourself). *Note: Avoid premade Jell-O snacks as many contain apple juice concentrate.*
- Broth without onion or garlic: try Gourmend Foods (chicken or beef broths), Rachel Pauls Happy Soup (bases for chicken, beef, or vegetable broth), Progresso reduced-sodium chicken broth, Savory Choice chicken broth packets (add hot water), or make your own.
- Beverages: water (plain or carbonated), Simply Lemonade (contains sugar, lemon juice), Gatorade (clear-liquid varieties made with sugar and dextrose; avoid red dyes, per hospital instructions), Clif Hydration Electrolyte Drink (lemon-lime flavor), tea, coffee, coconut water (keep portion to 3 ounces per serving). Try a half-and-half lemon-tea beverage: iced tea made with steeped green or black tea with a splash of Simply Lemonade and ice, or purchase a suitable premade version such as Honest Tea Half Tea & Half Lemonade.
- Hard candy (made with sugar, not high-fructose corn syrup): lemon drops (brand: Signature Select) or peppermint rounds (brand: YumEarth).
- Make-ahead frozen treat: fill a paper cup two-thirds full with Simply Lemonade or suitable Gatorade flavor; partially freeze for a slushy treat.

RESOURCES

Stay connected with Kate and Dr. Riehl!

Kate Scarlata's website: www.katescarlata.com
Dr. Riehl's website: www.drriehl.com
@MindYourGutOfficial on Instagram: Continue the
  learning, and participate in conversations regarding all
  things Mind Your Gut.
Scan the QR code to follow us at MindYourGutOfficial:

MIND YOUR GUT **THOUGHT RECORD**

Where are you? Who are you with?

What are your emotions or feelings?
Rate the intensity from 0–100.

Negative automatic thoughts:

Evidence that supports your thoughts:

Evidence that does not support your thoughts:

Alternative thought or helpful perspective:

Emotions or feelings in this moment.
Reconsider intensity from 0–100.

Figure 8. Mind Your Gut Thought Record

MIND YOUR GUT MY ESSENTIALS FOR HEALTH LIST

My favorite strategies:	Page #

Inhale...Exhale...

Figure 9. Mind Your Gut My Essentials for Health List

MIND YOUR GUT FOOD + LIFESTYLE TRACKER

TODAY'S DATE:

Breakfast	Lunch
Dinner	**Snacks**

HYDRATION *Please checkmark for each 8 oz fluid*

☐ ☐ ☐ ☐ ☐ ☐ ☐ ☐ ☐ ☐

BOWEL MOVEMENTS

EMOTIONS + MOOD

PHYSICAL SENSATIONS

MEDICINES + SUPPLEMENTS

MOVEMENT + JOY

MINDFUL RELAXATION

Figure 10. Mind Your Gut Food and Lifestyle Tracker

Bristol Stool Form Scale

Type 1		Separate hard lumps, like nuts
Type 2		Sausage shaped but lumpy
Type 3		Like a sausage but with cracks on the surface
Type 4		Like a sausage or snake, smooth and soft
Type 5		Soft blobs with clear-cut edges
Type 6		Fluffy pieces with ragged edges, a mushy stool
Type 7		Watery, no solid pieces

Figure 11. Bristol Stool Form Scale

LOW-FODMAP FOODS

Prepared Foods

Some brands work with outside companies to test for and certify the low-FODMAP content of their products. This certification makes it a bit easier for consumers to select low-FODMAP foods. The testing is done by two organizations: Monash University (in Melbourne, Australia) and FODMAP Friendly. But just because a product isn't certified doesn't mean it is *not* low-FODMAP. There are many food products made with low-FODMAP ingredients that you can enjoy.

Below you will find some of our favorite low-FODMAP-certified products. Note: Some companies do not certify all their products, so always check packaging and ingredients. And manufacturers can change ingredients at any time; this is another good reason to review the label of any product before consuming it.

Fody Foods provides a variety of delicious foods, all of which are certified low-FODMAP. Their product lineup includes salad dressings, garlic- and shallot-infused extra-virgin olive oil, pasta sauces, salsas, snack bars, and condiments such as ketchup, seasoning blends, marinades, and sauces. Fody takes the extra step to include gut-friendly ingredients, including extra-virgin olive oil, in many of their products.
www.fodyfoods.com

Schär, a well-known purveyor of gluten-free, celiac-friendly foods, has a number of products certified as low-FODMAP, including deli-style sourdough bread, deli-style seeded bread, ciabatta, multigrain ciabatta, baguette, pizza crust, Italian crostini, table crackers, rosemary table crackers, multigrain table crackers, entertainment crackers, Italian breadsticks, and crispbread.
www.schaer.com

BelliWelli offers a variety of low-FODMAP-certified baked snack bars with tempting flavors such as birthday cake, fudge brownie, blueberry muffin, and more.
www.belliwelli.com

COBS Bread offers low-FODMAP-certified breads and buns. Check out their LowFOD loaf, LowFOD mini loaf, or LowFOD bun.
www.cobsbread.com

Gourmend Foods offers low-FODMAP-certified organic chicken broth, garlic scape powder, garlic chive powder, garlic chive salt, green onion powder, and green onion salt.
www.gourmendfoods.com

Green Valley has a number of yogurt flavors that are certified low-FODMAP, including low-fat plain, vanilla, strawberry, and blueberry yogurts, and whole-milk plain yogurt. Other low-FODMAP-certified products include kefir, which comes in low-fat plain, whole-milk plain, and low-fat blueberry pomegranate acai. We also love their lactose-free cream cheese, sour cream, and cottage cheese.
www.greenvalleylactosefree.com

Bobo's offers a variety of certified-FODMAP-friendly oat-based bars and bites, including almond butter, banana chocolate chip, and more.
www.eatbobos.com

GoMacro sells dense and filling bars that are great for when you're on the go. The flavors that are certified low-FODMAP include mocha chocolate chip, banana and almond butter, dark chocolate and almond, peanut butter protein replenishment bar, sunflower and chocolate protein purity, coconut and almond butter and chocolate chips.
www.gomacro.com

Miracle Noodle offers a variety of low-carb and plant-based noodle options that are FODMAP-friendly certified.
www.miraclenoodle.com

San-J sells many gluten-free sauces and crackers that are also certified low-FODMAP. Gluten-free sauces that meet low-FODMAP specs include Szechuan sauce, tamari, lite tamari, reduced-sodium tamari, hoisin sauce, and Thai peanut sauce. Cracker options include tamari black sesame brown rice crackers, tamari brown sesame brown rice crackers, and sesame brown rice crackers.
www.san-j.com

ModifyHealth and **Epicured** both sell prepared low-FODMAP foods and meals delivered to your doorstep.
www.modifyhealth.com
www.epicured.com

Below you will find a few more of our favorite products made with low-FODMAP ingredients.

Baking Flours, Baking Mixes, Grains

Bob's Red Mill (www.bobsredmill.com)
  Gluten-free 1-to-1 baking flour
  White rice flour
  Oat flour
  Corn flour
  Polenta
  Rolled oats
  Steel-cut oats
  Oat bran

King Arthur (www.kingarthurbaking.com)

Gluten-free all-purpose flour
Gluten-free measure-for-measure flour
Gluten-free pancake mix

Namaste Foods (www.namastefoods.com)

Gluten-free Perfect Flour Blend
Organic yellow cake mix
Organic quick bread and muffin mix

Pizza Crusts, Pasta, Baked Snacks

Pizza crusts

Udi's gluten-free pizza crust, package of two
(www.udisglutenfree.com)
Schär gluten-free pizza crust (www.schaer.com)

Pasta

Barilla chickpea pasta (www.barilla.com)
Barilla gluten-free pasta (www.barilla.com)
Jovial organic brown rice pasta (https://jovialfoods.com)
Tinkyada brown rice pasta (www.tinkyada.com)

Snacks

Snyder's of Hanover: Gluten-free pretzel rods and
mini pretzels (www.snydersofhanover.com)
Lesser Evil Popcorn: Organic Avocado-Licious
(www.shop.lesserevil.com)
Blue Diamond: Almond Nut-Thins Hint of Sea Salt
(www.bluediamond.com)
Mary's Gone Crackers: Original
(www.shop.marysgonecrackers.com)

SUPPLEMENTS

Psyllium husk

> Konsyl Daily Psyllium Fiber (simply one ingredient)
> Kate Naturals Psyllium Husk Powder (can be used in baking)

Digestive enzymes (backed by science)*

> For symptoms of lactose intolerance: lactase enzyme supplement (select a brand that doesn't contain other FODMAP ingredients; we like Nature's Way)
> For IBS symptoms with ingestion of legumes and other higher-GOS foods: alpha-galactosidase (select a brand that doesn't contain other FODMAP ingredients; we like BeanAssist, by Enyzmedica, and Bean-zyme, by ValuePricedMeds)
> *For digestion of fructans, GOS and lactose, FODZYME may be trialed, but to date there are no studies in IBS. We are hopeful that work in this area will continue to emerge.

Peppermint oil (select enteric-coated)

> Pepogest (by Nature's Way) is our go-to
> IBgard is another option

Probiotic information (resources to help you find a probiotic backed by science to aid with particular symptoms or a diagnosis)

> International Scientific Association for Probiotics and Prebiotics: https://isappscience.org/
> Alliance for Education on Probiotics: https://aeprobio.com/
> Clinical Guide to US Probiotics (provides symptom- and diagnosis-based recommendations): www.usprobioticguide.com/PBCAdultHealth.html

DIAPHRAGMATIC BREATHING

For a helpful demonstration by Dr. Riehl, visit this website (or use the QR code):

www.youtube.com/watch?v=UB3tSaiEbNY

Also see Relaxation, Meditation, and Breathing Apps (below) for apps that teach diaphragmatic breathing.

MOOD AND ANXIETY SELF-SCREENING MEASURES

Anxiety Screening

GAD-7: https://screening.mhanational.org/screening-tools /anxiety/

Short Health Anxiety Inventory: https://psychology-tools.com /test/health-anxiety-inventory

Mood Screening

PHQ-9: https://screening.mhanational.org/screening-tools /depression/

SPECIALIZED HEALTH-CARE PROVIDERS

Finding a Gastroenterologist

American College of Gastroenterology:
https://gi.org/patients/find-a-gastroenterologist/

Mental Health Crisis Intervention

If you are having suicidal thoughts, we are especially concerned that you receive the support you need. We strongly urge you to contact one of the resources listed here:

- Call or text 988 for the Suicide & Crisis Lifeline (website: https://988lifeline.org)
- Veteran's Crisis Line: Dial 988, then press 1, or text 838255
- LGBTQ resources: Call the Trevor Lifeline at +1-866-488-7386, or text TREVOR to +1-202-304-1200

Finding a GI Psychologist or a General Mental Health Provider

When looking for a mental health professional to assist with the management of your IBS, ideally you will be able to find one who specializes in treating people with GI conditions. Alternatively, look for a licensed mental health provider with any of the following areas of expertise: health psychology, chronic illness, chronic pain, anxiety, depression, stress. You can also find a provider who specializes in evidence-based therapies such as cognitive-behavioral therapy, behavioral therapy, medical hypnotherapy, acceptance and commitment therapy, mindfulness-based stress reduction. The resources below can help:

Rome Foundation GastroPsych Clinician Directory:
https://romegipsych.org

GI Psychology:
www.gipsychology.com

Psychology Today Therapist Finder:
   www.psychologytoday.com/us/therapists
American Psychological Association:
   https://locator.apa.org
National Register of Health Service Psychologists:
   www.findapsychologist.org
Association for Behavioral and Cognitive Therapies:
   www.findcbt.org

Finding a Provider for Gut-Directed Hypnotherapy

IBSHypnosis.com, a public information website
operated by Dr. Olafur Palsson:
https://ibshypnosis.com/IBSclinicians.html

Finding a Pain Psychologist

American Association of Pain Psychology Provider Directory:
https://aapainpsychology.org/find-a-provider/#!directory
/map/ord=lnm

Finding an Eating Disorder Specialist

Multi-Service Eating Disorders Association:
   www.medainc.org
National Alliance for Eating Disorders:
   www.allianceforeatingdisorders.com
National Eating Disorders Association (NEDA) Online
   Treatment Provider Database:
   www.nationaleatingdisorders.org/find-treatment
Psychology Today Eating Disorder Specialist Directory:
   www.psychologytoday.com/us/therapists/eating-disorders

Finding a Low-FODMAP Expert Dietitian

A number of online resources can help you find a dietitian with
expertise in the low-FODMAP diet. We recommend the following:

Kate Scarlata's FODMAP dietitian registry:
www.katescarlata.com (search under the "FODMAP
Resources" tab)

Monash University: www.monashfodmap.com (click on "Find
a Dietitian" for a worldwide directory of dietitians who have
successfully completed Monash's FODMAP course)

Academy of Nutrition and Dietetics: www.eatright.org (click
on "Find a Nutrition Expert," and enter your zip code for a
directory of registered dietitians in your area; you can sort
the list by specialty, including "Gluten Intolerance-
Digestive Health-GI Disorders," "Food Allergies and
Intolerances," etc.)

The American Gastroenterological Association is currently
working on a GI expert dietitian listing; stay tuned at
www.gastro.org

MISCELLANEOUS RESOURCES

Intuitive Eating

Website: www.intuitiveeating.org

Book: *Intuitive Eating: A Revolutionary Anti-Diet Approach*
(4th edition) by Evelyn Tribole and Elyse Resch

Pelvic Floor Physical Therapy

Pelvic floor physical therapy is a subspecialty of physical therapy
that concentrates on dysfunction of the pelvic floor muscles, pain,
and weakness. It can be especially helpful for some IBS patients
with either constipation or diarrhea, as well as those with urinary or
reproductive issues. Speak with a physician about whether you are a
candidate for this form of treatment.

Consult the following resources to learn more about this type of
physical therapy and locate a therapist:

Where to find a pelvic floor PT in your area:
    https://pelvicguru.com/directory/
Herman Wallace: https://hermanwallace.com/
Academy of Pelvic Health Physical Therapy:
    https://aptapelvichealth.org

Toilet Accessories

Comfort is key when it comes to using the toilet. We recommend the following accessories:
    Squatty Potty: www.squattypotty.com
    Tushy Bidet: www.hellotushy.com

Proper Pooping Position

Position matters when you're trying to poop! Figure 12 shows the proper position to allow for easier release of stool.

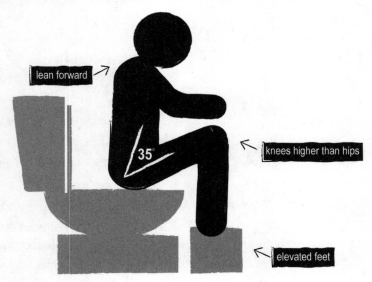

Figure 12. Proper Pooping Position

The makers of the Squatty Potty offer lots of pooping info: www.squattypotty.com.

MORE IBS-RELATED APPS AND WEBSITES

Hypnotherapy and Behavioral Health Apps and Websites

These science-backed digital resources can provide you with tools, strategies, and relief. Note that many require some out-of-pocket cost.

Nerva provides science-based hypnotherapy via a smartphone app. The program is designed to help correct the miscommunication that often occurs in IBS between the gut and the brain. The six-week program requires about fifteen minutes per day. https://try.nervaibs.com

Regulora is the first FDA-approved treatment for IBS abdominal pain in adults. The mobile app offers seven thirty-minute sessions of virtual behavioral therapy over three months. The sessions, based on an evidence-based gut-directed hypnotherapy protocol, require a prescription from your health-care provider. www.regulorahcp.com

Mahana Therapeutics offers a digital app that delivers a three-month program for adults with IBS using cognitive-behavioral therapy to ease IBS symptoms and to help users develop new IBS-management skills and habits. Users receive customized feedback through tracking of IBS symptoms, mental health, and physical health. The program requires just a ten-minute commitment per day. www.mahana.com

Trellus Health is a digital health company that provides behavioral health curricula utilizing evidence-based psychological strategies to aid with the management of IBS. (Also available for people with inflammatory bowel disease.) The Trellus Elevate virtual support program is available for both patients and their health-care providers. Access to a care navigator or registered dietitian is also available. www.trellushealth.com

In-Home Yoga and Exercise Apps and Websites

Yoga International: www.yogainternational.com (search "5 Yoga Poses for IBS")

GI-focused yoga and breathing interventions led by Gina Norman with Kaia Yoga: https://giresearchfoundation.org/yoga-breathing-and-meditation/

SarahBethYoga: Search "SarahBethYoga" on YouTube. She offers a wide range of free yoga practices ranging from five to thirty minutes, including some targeted to promote good digestion

Glo (at-home classes in yoga, meditation, fitness, and Pilates): www.glo.com

Walk at Home with Lesli Sansone (a full-body, walking-based exercise program that you can do in your home): walkathome.com

Low-FODMAP Diet Apps

Monash University FODMAP Diet app: www.monashfodmap.com/ibs-central/i-have-ibs/get-the-app

FODMAP Friendly app: https://fodmapfriendly.com/app

Relaxation, Meditation, and Breathing Apps

Search for these by name in your favorite app store.

Calm
Headspace
Mindfulness Coach
Buddhify
Insight Timer
Breethe
Christian + Meditation
BellyBio Interactive Breathing (diaphragmatic breathing)
Breathe2Relax (diaphragmatic breathing)

IBS Symptom- and Lifestyle-Tracking Apps

Search for these by name in your favorite app store.

> My GI Health GI Symptom Tracker
> My IBS Symptom & Health Diary
> Cara Care: IBS, FODMAP Tracker
> Bowelle: The IBS Tracker
> Constipation Diary
> Fig: Food Scanner (also see www.foodisgood.com)

Bathroom Locator Apps

Search for these by name in your favorite app store.

> Flush: Toilet Finder & Map
> We Can't Wait: Restroom Finder

IBS Patient Support Apps and Websites

The following websites offer updates on IBS-related research, webinars, podcasts, and additional support for living well with IBS.

> GI OnDemand: https://giondemand.com
> GastroGirl: https://gastrogirl.com
> IBS Patient Support Group: www.ibspatient.org
> Tuesday Night IBS: www.tuesdaynightibs.com
> International Foundation for Gastrointestinal Disorders:
>   https://iffgd.org
> Rome Foundation: https://theromefoundation.org

VIRTUAL REALITY FOR IBS

Virtual reality (VR) technology provides an immersive, multi-sensory, and three-dimensional (3D) environment that enables users to have modified experiences of reality and be engaged in the present. SynerGI (formerly IBS VR) provides a "virtual clinic" experience using the latest VR technology and science to allow users to practice behavioral techniques for the management of IBS. The goal of SynerGI is to strengthen the brain-gut axis to improve quality of life.

SynerGI informational video:
    https://virtualmedicine.org/synergi
VR apps recommended by Cedars-Sinai Virtual
    Medicine Program:
    https://virtualmedicine.org/favorite_vr

REFERENCES

CHAPTER 1

American Academy of Allergy, Asthma, and Immunology. "Food allergy versus food intolerance." Accessed September 8, 2023. http://www.aaaai .org/aaaai/media/medialibrary/pdf%20Documents/Libraries/EL-food -allergies-vs-intolerance-patient.pdf.

Barrett, Jacqueline S. "How to institute the low-FODMAP diet." *Journal of Gastroenterology and Hepatology* 32, no. 1 (March 2017):8–10. doi: 10.1111 /jgh.13686.

Basnayake, Chamara, Michael A. Kamm, Annalise Stanley, Amy Wilson-O'Brien, Kathryn Burrell, Isabella Lees-Trinca, Angela Khera, et al. "Standard gastroenterologist versus multidisciplinary treatment for functional gastrointestinal disorders (MANTRA): an open-label, single-centre, randomised controlled trial." *Lancet Gastroenterology and Hepatology* 5, no. 10 (October 2020):890–899. doi: 10.1016/S2468-1253(20)30215-6.

Black, Christopher J., Heidi M. Staudacher, Alexander C. Ford. "Efficacy of a low FODMAP diet in irritable bowel syndrome: systematic review and network meta-analysis." *Gut* 71, no. 6 (June 2022):1117–1126. doi: 10.1136 /gutjnl-2021-325214.

Black, Christopher J., Elyse R. Thakur, Lesley A. Houghton, Eamonn M. M. Quigley, Paul Moayyedi, Alexander C. Ford. "Efficacy of psychological therapies for irritable bowel syndrome: systematic review and network meta-analysis." *Gut* 69, no. 8 (August 2020):1441–1451. doi: 10.1136 /gutjnl-2020-321191.

Böhn, Lena, Stine Störsrud, Hans Törnblom, Ulf Bengtsson, Magnus Simrén. "Self-reported food-related gastrointestinal symptoms in IBS are common and associated with more severe symptoms and reduced quality of life." *American Journal of Gastroenterology* 108, no. 5 (May 2013):634–641. doi: 10.1038/ajg.2013.105.

Chang, Lin. "Brain-gut interactions in IBS: novel applications for clinical practice." Morton I. Grossman Distinguished Lectureship, presented at American Gastroenterological Association's Digestive Disease Week, Chicago, IL, May 2023.

Chey, William D., Laurie Keefer, Kevin Whelan, Peter R. Gibson. "Behavioral and diet therapies in integrated care for patients with irritable bowel syndrome." *Gastroenterology* 160, no. 1 (January 2021):47–62. doi: 10.1053/j.gastro.2020.06.099.

Cohen, Stanley A. "The clinical consequences of sucrase-isomaltase deficiency." *Molecular and Cellular Pediatrics* 3, no. 1 (2016):5. doi:10.1186 /s40348-015-0028-0.

Diehl, D. J., S. Gershon. "The role of dopamine in mood disorders." *Comprehensive Psychiatry* 33, no. 2 (March–April 1992):115–120. doi: 10.1016/0010-440x(92)90007-d.

Dorfman, Lev, Anundorn Wongteerasut, Khalil El-Chammas, Rashmi Sahay, Lin Fei, Ajay Kaul. "Novel sensory trigger for gastrocolonic response." *Journal of Neurogastroenterology and Motility*. Epub ahead of print (January 2023):e14528. doi: 10.1111/nmo.14528.

Drossman, Doug A. "Functional gastrointestinal disorders: history, pathophysiology, clinical features and Rome IV." *Gastroenterology* 150, no. 6 (May 2016):1262–1279. doi: 10.1053/j.gastro.2016.02.032.

Eswaran, Shanti L., William D. Chey, Theresa Han-Markeym, Sara Ball, Kenya Jackson. "A randomized controlled trial comparing the low FODMAP diet vs. modified NICE guidelines in US adults with IBS-D." *American Journal of Gastroenterology* 111, no. 12 (December 2016):1824–1832. doi: 10.1038/ajg.2016.434.

Eswaran, Shanti, Jane Muir, William D. Chey. "Fiber and functional gastrointestinal disorders." *American Journal of Gastroenterology* 108, no. 5 (May 2013):718–727. doi: 10.1038/ajg.2013.63.

Ford, Alexander C., Ami D. Sperber, Maura Corsetti, Michael Camilleri. "Irritable bowel syndrome." *The Lancet* 396, no. 10263 (November 2020):1675–1688. doi: 10.1016/S0140-6736(20)31548-8.

Goldstein, Ryan S., Brooks D. Cash. "Making a confident diagnosis of irritable bowel syndrome." *Gastroenterology Clinics of North America* 50, no. 3 (September 2021):547–563. doi: 10.1016/j.gtc.2021.03.004.

Henström, Maria, Lena Diekmann, Ferdinando Bonfiglio, Fatemeh Hadizadeh, Eva-Maria Kuech, Maren von Kockritz-Blickwede, Louise B. Thingholm, et al. "Functional variants in the sucrase-isomaltase gene associate with increased risk of irritable bowel syndrome." *Gut* 67, no. 2 (February 2018):263–270. doi: 10.1136/gutjnl-2016-312456.

Jianqin, Sun, Xu Leiming, Xia Lu, Gregory W. Yelland, Jiayi Ni, Andrew Clarke. "Effects of milk containing only A2 beta casein versus milk containing both A1 and A2 beta casein proteins on gastrointestinal physiology, symptoms of discomfort, and cognitive behavior of people with self-reported intolerance to traditional cows' milk." *Nutrition Journal* 15, no. 1 (April 2016):45. doi: 10.1186/s12937-016-0147-z.

Keefer, Laurie, Olafur S. Palsson, John E. Pandolfino. "Best practice update: incorporating psychogastroenterology into management of digestive disorders." *Gastroenterology* 154, no. 5 (April 2018):1249–1257. doi: 10.1053/j.gastro.2018.01.045.

Lacy, Brian E., Mark Pimentel, Darren M. Brenner, William D. Chey, Laurie A. Keefer, Millie D. Long, Baha Moshiree. "ACG clinical guideline: management of irritable bowel syndrome." *American Journal of Gastroenterology* 116, no. 1 (January 2021):17–44. doi: 10.14309/ajg.0000000000001036.

Mayer, Emeran, Hyo Jin Ryu, Ravi R. Bhatt. "The neurobiology of irritable bowel syndrome." *Molecular Psychiatry*. Epub ahead of print (February 2023). doi: 10.1038/s41380-023-01972-w.

Melchior, Chloe, Joost Algera, Esther Colomier, Hans Törnblom, Magnus Simrén, Stine Störsrud. "Food avoidance and restriction in irritable bowel syndrome: relevance for symptoms, quality of life and nutrient intake." *Clinical Gastroenterology and Hepatology* 20, no. 6 (June 2022):1290–1298. e4. doi: 10.1016/j.cgh.2021.07.004.

Murray, Helen B., Bethany Doerfler, Kimberly N. Harer, Laurie Keefer. "Psychological considerations in the dietary management of patients with DGBI." *American Journal of Gastroenterology* 117, no. 6 (June 2022):985–994. doi: 10.14309/ajg.0000000000001766.

Oka, Priya, Heather Parr, Brigida Barberio, Christopher J. Black, Edoardo V. Savarino, Alexander C. Ford. "Global prevalence of irritable bowel syndrome according to Rome III or IV criteria: a systematic review and meta-analysis." *Lancet Gastroenterology and Hepatology* 5, no. 10 (October 2020): 908–917. doi: 10.1016/S2468-1253(20)30217-X. Erratum in: *Lancet Gastroenterology and Hepatology* 5, no. 12 (December 2020):e8.

Ortolani, Claudio, Elide A. Pastorello. "Food allergies and food intolerances." *Best Practice and Research Clinical Gastroenterology* 20, no. 3 (2006):467–483. doi: 10.1016/j.bpg.2005.11.010.

Palsson, Olafur S., William Whitehead, Hans Törnblom, Ami D. Sperber, Magnus Simren. "Prevalence of Rome IV functional bowel disorders among adults in the United States, Canada, and the United Kingdom." *Gastroenterology* 158, no. 5 (April 2020):1262–1273. doi: 10.1053/j.gastro.2019.12.021.

Pellissier, Sonia, Bruno Bonaz. "The place of stress and emotions in the irritable bowel syndrome." *Vitamins and Hormones* no. 103 (2017):327–354. doi: 10.1016/bs.vh.2016.09.005.

Rosell-Camps, Antonio, Sara Zibetti, Gerardo Pérez-Esteban, Magdalena Vila-Vidal, Laia Ferrés-Ramis, Elisa García-Teresa-García. "Histamine intolerance as a cause of chronic digestive complaints in pediatric patients." *Revista Espanola De Enfermedades Digestivas* 105, no. 4 (April 2013):201–206. doi: 10.4321/s1130-01082013000400004.

Staudacher, Heidi M., Sophie Mahoney, Kim Canale, Daniel So, Amy Lough-man, Rachelle Opie, Lauren Beswick, Chris Hair, Felice Jacka. "A Medi-terranean diet is feasible in patients with irritable bowel syndrome: a pilot randomized controlled trial." Presented at American Gastroenterological Association's Digestive Disease Week, Chicago, IL, May 2023.

CHAPTER 2

Black, Christopher J., Elyse R. Thakur, Lesley A. Houghton, Eamonn M. M. Quigley, Paul Moayyedi, Alexander C. Ford. "Efficacy of psycholog-ical therapies for irritable bowel syndrome: systematic review and net-work meta-analysis." *Gut* 69, no. 8 (August 2020):1441–1451. doi: 10.1136 /gutjnl-2020-321191.

Black, Christopher J., Alexander C. Ford. "Global burden of irritable bowel syndrome: trends, predictions and risk factors." *Nature Review Gas-troenterology Hepatology* 17, no. 8 (August 2020):473–486. doi: 10.1038 /s41575-020-0286-8.

Burton Murray, Helen, Brjánn Ljótsson. "Future of brain-gut behavior thera-pies: mediators and moderators." *Gastroenterology Clinics of North America* 51, no. 4 (December 2022):723–739. doi: 10.1016/j.gtc.2022.06.011.

Clauw, Daniel J., George P. Chrousos. "Chronic pain and fatigue syndromes: overlapping clinical and neuroendocrine features and potential patho-genic mechanisms." *Neuroimmunomodulation* 4, no. 3 (1997):134–153. doi: 10.1159/000097332.

Drossman, Douglas A., Carolyn B. Morris, Susan Schneck, Yuming J. Hu, Nancy J. Norton, William F. Norton, Stephan Weinland, et al. "Inter-national survey of patients with IBS: symptom features and their severity, health status, treatments, and risk taking to achieve clinical benefit." *Jour-nal of Clinical Gastroenterology* 43, no. 6 (July 2009):541–550. doi: 10.1097 /MCG.0b013e318189a7f9.

Farzaei, Mohammad H., Roodabeh Bahramsoltani, Mohammad Abdollahi, Roja Rahimi. "The role of visceral hypersensitivity in irritable bowel syndrome: pharmacological targets and novel treatments." *Journal of Neurogastroenterology and Motility* 22, no. 4 (October 2016):558–574. doi: 10.5056/jnm16001.

Halland, Magnus, Adil E. Bharucha, Michael D. Crowell, Karthik Ravi, David A. Katzka. "Effects of diaphragmatic breathing on the pathophys-iology and treatment of upright gastroesophageal reflux: a randomized controlled trial." *American Journal of Gastroenterology* 116, no. 1 (January 2021):86–94. doi: 10.14309/ajg.0000000000000913.

Harris, Russ. *The single most powerful technique for extreme fusion.* 2016. www.actmindfully.com.au/upimages/The_Single_Most_Powerful _Technique_for_Extreme_Fusion_-_Russ_Harris_-_October_2016.pdf.

Hazlett-Stevens, Holly, Michelle G. Craske, Emeran A. Mayer, Lin Chang, Bruce D. Naliboff. "Prevalence of irritable bowel syndrome among university students: the roles of worry, neuroticism, anxiety sensitivity and visceral anxiety." *Journal of Psychosomatic Research* 55, no. 6 (December 2003):501–505. doi: 10.1016/s0022-3999(03)00019-9.

Karantanos, Theodoros, Theofano Markoutsaki, Maria Gazouli, Nicholas P. Anagnou, Dimitrios G. Karamanolis. "Current insights into the pathophysiology of irritable bowel syndrome." *Gut Pathogens* 2, no. 1 (May 2010):3. doi: 10.1186/1757-4749-2-3.

Kinsinger, Sarah W. "Cognitive-behavioral therapy for patients with irritable bowel syndrome: current insights." *Psychology Research and Behavior Management* no. 10 (July 2017):231–237. doi: 10.2147/PRBM.S120817.

Konturek, Peter C., T. Brzozowski, S. J. Konturek. "Stress and the gut: pathophysiology, clinical consequences, diagnostic approach and treatment options." *Journal of Physiology and Pharmacology* 62, no. 6 (December 2011):591–599. PMID: 22314561.

Labus, Jennifer S., R. Bolus, L. Chang, I. Wiklund, J. Naesdal, E. A. Mayer, B. D. Naliboff. "The visceral sensitivity index: development and validation of a gastrointestinal symptom-specific anxiety scale." *Alimentary Pharmacology and Therapeutics* 20, no. 1 (July 2004):89–97. doi: 10.1111/j.1365-2036.2004.02007.x.

Labus, Jennifer S., Emeran A. Mayer, Lin Chang, Rodger Bolus, Bruce D. Naliboff. "The central role of gastrointestinal-specific anxiety in irritable bowel syndrome: further validation of the visceral sensitivity index." *Psychosomatic Medicine* 69, no. 1 (January 2007):89–98. doi: 10.1097/PSY.0b013e31802e2f24.

Lacy, Brian E., Kelly K. Everhart, Kirsten T. Weiser, Ryan DeLee, Sebastian Strobel, Corey Siegel, Michael D. Crowell. "IBS patients' willingness to take risks with medications." *American Journal of Gastroenterology* 107, no. 6 (June 2012):804–809. doi: 10.1038/ajg.2011.485.

Lally, Phillippa, Cornelia H. M. van Jaarsveld, Henry W. W. Potts, Jane Wardle. "How are habits formed: modelling habit formation in the real world." *European Journal of Social Psychology* 40, no. 6 (October 2009):998–1009. doi: 10.1002/ejsp.674.

Lee, Anna H., Swapna Mahurkar-Joshi, Bruce D. Naliboff, Wendi G. LeBrett, Jennifer S. Lubus, Arpana Gupta, Kirsten Tillisch, Emeran A. Mayer, Lin Chang. "Sex difference in adverse childhood experiences and their effect on IBS status and resilience." Presented at American Gastroenterological Association's Digestive Disease Week, Chicago, IL, May 2023.

Ludidi, S., J. M. Conchillo, D. Keszthelyi, M. Van Avesaat, J. W. Kruimel, D. M. Jonkers, A. A. Masclee. "Rectal hypersensitivity as hallmark for irritable bowel syndrome: defining the optimal cutoff." *Journal of Neurogastroenterology and Motility* 24, no. 8 (August 2012):729–733, e345–6. doi: 10.1111/j.1365-2982.2012.01926.x.

Madison, Annelise, Janice K. Kiecolt-Glaser. "Stress, depression, diet, and the gut microbiota: human-bacteria interactions at the core of psychoneuroimmunology and nutrition." *Current Opinions in Behavioral Sciences* 28, (August 2019):105–110. doi: 10.1016/j.cobeha.2019.01.011.

Mao, Gen Xiang, Xiao Guang Lan, Yong Bao Cao, Zhuo Mei Chen, Zhi Hua He, Yuan Dong Lv, Ya Zhen Wang, et al. "Effects of short-term forest bathing on human health in a broad-leaved evergreen forest in Zhejiang Province, China." *Biomedical and Environmental Sciences* 25, no. 3 (June 2012):317–324. doi: 10.3967/0895-3988.2012.03.010.

Mayer, Emeran, Hyo Jin Ryu, Ravi R. Bhatt. "The neurobiology of irritable bowel syndrome." *Molecular Psychiatry*. Epub ahead of print (February 2023). doi: 10.1038/s41380-023-01972-w.

Oschman, James L., Gaetan Chevalier, Richard Brown. "The effects of grounding (earthing) on inflammation, the immune response, wound healing, and prevention and treatment of chronic inflammatory and autoimmune diseases." *Journal of Inflammation Research* 24, no. 8 (March 2015):83–96. doi: 10.2147/JIR.S69656.

Qin, Hong-Yan, Chung-Wah Cheng, Xu-Dong Tang, Zhao-Xiang Bian. "Impact of psychological stress on irritable bowel syndrome." *World Journal of Gastroenterology* 20, no. 39 (October 2014):14126–14131. doi: 10.3748/wjg.v20.i39.14126.

Riehl, Megan E., Jami A. Kinnucan, William D. Chey, Ryan W. Stidham. "Nuances of the psychogastroenterology patient: a predictive model for gastrointestinal quality of life improvement." *Journal of Neurogastroenterology and Motility* 31, no. 9 (September 2019):e13663. doi: 10.1111/nmo.13663.

Simrén, Magnus, Hans Törnblom, Olafur S. Palsson, Miranda A. L. van Tilburg, Lukas Van Oudenhove, Jan Tack, William E. Whitehead. "Visceral hypersensitivity is associated with GI symptom severity in functional GI disorders: consistent findings from five different patient cohorts." *Gut* 67, no. 2 (February 2018):255–262. doi: 10.1136/gutjnl-2016-312361.

Sugaya, Nagisa, Kentaro Shirotsuki, Mutsuhiro Nakao. "Cognitive behavioral treatment for irritable bowel syndrome: a recent literature review." *BioPsychoSocial Medicine* 15, no. 1 (November 2021):23. doi: 10.1186/s13030-021-00226-x.

Ziadni, Maisa S., Dokyoung S. You, Lucia Johnson, Mark A. Lumley, Beth D. Darnall. "Emotions matter: the role of emotional approach coping in chronic pain." *European Journal of Pain* 24, no. 9 (October 2020):1775–1784. doi: 10.1002/ejp.1625.

CHAPTER 3

Addante, Raymond, Bruce Naliboff, Wendy Shih, Angela P. Presson, Kirsten Tillisch, Emeran A. Mayer, Lin Chang. "Predictors of health-related quality of life in irritable bowel syndrome patients compared with healthy individuals." *Journal of Clinical Gastroenterology* 53, no. 4 (April 2019):e142–e149. doi: 10.1097/MCG.0000000000000978.

Böhn, Lena, Stine Störsrud, Hans Törnblom, Ulf Bengtsson, Magnus Simrén. "Self-reported food-related gastrointestinal symptoms in IBS are common and associated with more severe symptoms and reduced quality of life." *American Journal of Gastroenterology* 108, no. 5 (May 2013):634–641. doi: 10.1038/ajg.2013.105.

Carney, Colleen, Rachel Manber. *Quiet Your Mind and Get to Sleep: Solutions to Insomnia for Those with Depression, Anxiety, or Chronic Pain.* Oakland, CA: New Harbinger Publications, 2009.

Carney, Colleen, Rachel Waters. "Constructive worry instructions." Website of Colleen Carney, 2006. https://drcolleencarney.com/wp-content/uploads/2013/05/Constructive-Worry-Worksheet.pdf.

Cheng, C., W. Hui, S. Lam. "Perceptual style and behavioral pattern of individuals with functional gastrointestinal disorders." *Health Psychology Journal* 19, no. 2 (March 2000):146–154. doi: 10.1037//0278-6133.19.2.146.

Craske, Michelle G., Kate B. Wolitzky-Taylor, Jennifer Labus, Stephen Wu, Michael Frese, Emeran A. Mayer, Bruce D. Naliboff. "A cognitive-behavioral treatment for irritable bowel syndrome using interoceptive exposure to visceral sensations." *Behaviour Research and Therapy* 49, no. 6–7 (June 2011):413–421. doi: 10.1016/j.brat.2011.04.001.

Hunt, Melissa G. "Cognitive-behavioral therapy for irritable bowel syndrome." In *Using Central Neuromodulators and Psychological Therapies to Manage Patients with Disorders of Gut-Brain Interaction*, edited by W. Harley Sobin, 95–141. Cham, Switzerland: Springer, 2019.

Jacobs, Jonathan P., Arpana Gupta, Ravi R. Bhatt, Jacob Brawer, Kan Gao, Kirsten Tillisch, Venu Lagishetty, et al. "Cognitive behavioral therapy for irritable bowel syndrome induces bidirectional alterations in the brain-gut-microbiome axis associated with gastrointestinal symptom improvement." *Microbiome* 9, no. 1 (November 2021):236. doi: 10.1186/s40168-021-01188-6.

Naliboff, Bruce D., Suzanne R. Smith, John G. Serpa, Kelsey T. Laird, Jean Stains, Lynn S. Connolly, Jennifer S. Labus, et al. "Mindfulness-based stress reduction improves irritable bowel syndrome (IBS) symptoms via specific aspects of mindfulness." *Journal of Neurogastroenterology and Motility* 32, no. 9 (September 2020):e13828. doi: 10.1111/nmo.13828.

Nee, Judy, Anthony Lembo. "Review article: current and future treatment approaches for IBS with diarrhoea (IBS-D) and IBS mixed pattern (IBS-M)." *Alimentary Pharmacology and Therapeutics* 54, Suppl. 1 (December 2021):S63–S74. doi: 10.1111/apt.16625.

Paine, Peter. "Review article: current and future treatment approaches for pain in IBS." *Alimentary Pharmacology and Therapeutics* 54, Suppl. 1 (December 2021):S75–S88. doi: 10.1111/apt.16550.

CHAPTER 4

Cascio, Christopher N., Matthew B. O'Donnell, Francis J. Tinney, Matthew D. Lieberman, Shelley E. Taylor, Victor J. Strecher, Emily B. Falk. "Self-affirmation activates brain systems associated with self-related processing and reward and is reinforced by future orientation." *Social Cognitive and Affective Neuroscience* 11, no. 4 (April 2016):621–629. doi: 10.1093/scan/nsv136.

Cohen, Geoffrey L., David K. Sherman. "The psychology of change: self-affirmation and social psychological intervention." *Annual Review of Psychology* 65 (2014):333–371. doi: 10.1146/annurev-psych-010213-115137.

Dishman, Rod K., Hans-Rudolf Berthoud, Frank W. Booth, Carl W. Cotman, V. Reggie Edgerton, Monika R. Fleshner, Simon C. Gandevia, et al. "Neurobiology of exercise." *Obesity (Silver Spring)* 14, no. 3 (March 2006):345–356. doi: 10.1038/oby.2006.46.

D'Silva, Adrijana, Deborah A. Marshall, Jeffrey Vallance, Yasmin Nasser, Vidya Rajagopalan, Gail MacKean, Maitreyi Raman. "Meditation and yoga for irritable bowel syndrome: study protocol for a randomised clinical trial (MY-IBS study)." *BMJ Open* 12, no. 5 (May 2022):e059604. doi: 10.1136/bmjopen-2021-059604.

Elkins, Gary R., R. Lynae Roberts, Lauren Simicich. "Mindful self-hypnosis for self-care: an integrative model and illustrative case example." *American Journal of Clinical Hypnosis* 61, no. 1 (July 2018):45–56. doi: 10.1080/00029157.2018.1456896.

Herring, Matthew P., Timothy W. Puetz, Patrick J. O'Connor, Rodney K. Dishman. "Effect of exercise training on depressive symptoms among patients with a chronic illness: a systematic review and meta-analysis of randomized controlled trials." *Archives of Internal Medicine* 172, no. 2 (January 2012):101–111. doi: 10.1001/archinternmed.2011.696.

Johannesson, Elisabet, Gisela Ringström, Hasse Abrahamsson, Riadh Sadik. "Intervention to increase physical activity in irritable bowel syndrome shows long-term positive effects." *World Journal of Gastroenterology* 21, no. 2 (January 2015):600–608. doi: 10.3748/wjg.v21.i2.600.

Johannesson, Elisabet, Magnus Simrén, Hans Strid, Antal Bajor, Riadh Sadik. "Physical activity improves symptoms in irritable bowel syndrome: a randomized controlled trial." *American Journal of Gastroenterology* 106, no. 5 (May 2011):915–922. doi: 10.1038/ajg.2010.480.

Kavuri, Vijaya, Nagarathna Raghuram, Ariel Malamud, Senthamil R. Selvan. "Irritable bowel syndrome: yoga as remedial therapy." *Evidence-Based Complementary and Alternative Medicine* (2015):398156. doi: 10.1155/2015/398156.

Lowén, Mats B. O., Emeran A. Mayer, Martha Sjöberg, Kirsten Tillisch, Bruce Naliboff, Jennifer Labus, Peter Lundberg, et al. "Effect of hypnotherapy and educational intervention on brain response to visceral stimulus in the irritable bowel syndrome." *Alimentary Pharmacology and Therapeutics* 37, no. 12 (June 2013):1184–1197. doi: 10.1111/apt.12319.

Palsson, Olafur S., Sarah Ballou. "Hypnosis and cognitive behavioral therapies for the management of gastrointestinal disorders." *Current Gastroenterology Reports* 22, no. 7 (June 2020):31. doi: 10.1007/s11894-020-00769-z.

Palsson, Olafur S. "Hypnosis treatment of gastrointestinal disorders: a comprehensive review of the empirical evidence." *American Journal of Clinical Hypnosis* 58, no. 2 (October 2015):134–158. doi: 10.1080/00029157 .2015.1039114.

Patel, Nihal, Brian Lacy. "Does yoga help patients with irritable bowel syndrome?," *Clinical Gastroenterology and Hepatology* 14, no. 12 (December 2016):1732–1734. doi: 10.1016/j.cgh.2016.08.014.

Peters, Simone, Peter Gibson, Emma Halmos. "App-delivered gut-directed hypnotherapy program Nerva improves symptoms in patients with irritable bowel syndrome, but how can we ensure users are compliant?," *American College of Gastroenterology 2022 Annual Scientific Meeting Abstracts*. Charlotte, NC: American College of Gastroenterology, 2022.

Posserud, I., P. Agerforz, R. Ekman, E. S. Björnsson, H. Abrahamsson, M. Simrén. "Altered visceral perceptual and neuroendocrine response in patients with irritable bowel syndrome during mental stress." *Gut* 53, no. 8 (August 2004):1102–1108. doi: 10.1136/gut.2003.017962.

Schumann, Dania, Dennis Anheyer, Romy Lauche, Gustav Dobos, Jost Langhorst, Holger Cramer. "Effect of yoga in the therapy of irritable bowel syndrome: a systematic review." *Clinical Gastroenterology and Hepatology* 14, no. 12 (December 2016):1720–1731. doi: 10.1016/j.cgh.2016.04.026.

Shah, Khushbu, Maria Ramos-Garcia, Jay Bhavsar, Paul Lehrer. "Mind-body treatments of irritable bowel syndrome symptoms: an updated meta-analysis." *Behaviour Research and Therapy* 128 (May 2020):103462. doi: 10.1016/j.brat.2019.103462.

Shinozaki, Masae, Motoyori Kanazawa, Michiko Kano, Yuka End, Naoki Nakaya, Michio Hongo, Shin Fukudo. "Effect of autogenic training on general improvement in patients with irritable bowel syndrome: a randomized controlled trial." *Applied Psychophysiology and Biofeedback* 35, no. 3 (September 2010):189–198. doi: 10.1007/s10484-009-9125-y.

Slonena, Elizabeth E., Gary R. Elkins. "Effects of a brief mindful hypnosis intervention on stress reactivity: a randomized active control study." *International Journal of Clinical and Experimental Hypnosis* 69, no. 4 (October–December 2021):453–467. doi: 10.1080/00207144.2021.1952845.

Steele, Claude M. "The psychology of self-affirmation: sustaining the integrity of the self." *Advances in Experimental Social Psychology* 21, no. 2 (1988): 261–302.

Vasant, Dipesh H., Peter J. Whorwell. "Gut-focused hypnotherapy for functional gastrointestinal disorders: evidence-based, practical aspects, and the Manchester Protocol." *Neurogastroenterology and Motility* 31, no. 8 (August 2019):e13573. doi: 10.1111/nmo.13573.

CHAPTER 5

Armstrong, Heather, Interdeep Mander, Zhengxiao Zhang, David Armstrong, Eytan Wine. "Not all fibers are born equal: variable response to dietary fiber subtypes in IBD." *Frontiers in Pediatrics* 15, no. 8 (January 2021):620189. doi: 10.3389/fped.2020.620189.

Böhn, Lena, Stine Störsrud, Hans Törnblom, Ulf Bengtsson, Magnus Simrén. "Self-reported food-related gastrointestinal symptoms in IBS are common and associated with more severe symptoms and reduced quality of life." *American Journal of Gastroenterology* 108, no. 5 (May 2013):634–641. doi: 10.1038/ajg.2013.105.

Brown, S. R., P. A. Cann, N. W. Read. "Effect of coffee on distal colon function." *Gut* 31, no. 4 (April 1990):450–453. doi: 10.1136/gut.31.4.450.

Esmaillzadeh, Ahmad, Ammar H. Keshteli, Maryan Hajishafiee, Awat Feizi, Christine Feinle-Bisset, Peyman Adibi. "Consumption of spicy foods and the prevalence of irritable bowel syndrome." *World Journal of Gastroenterology* 19, no. 38 (October 2013):6465–6471. doi: 10.3748/wjg.v19.i38.6465.

Halmos, Emma P., Peter R. Gibson. "Controversies and reality of the FODMAP diet for patients with irritable bowel syndrome." *Journal of Gastroenterology and Hepatology* 34, no. 7 (July 2019):1134–1142. doi: 10.1111/jgh.14650.

Iriondo-DeHond, Amaia, Jose A. Uranga, Maria D. Del Castrillo, Raquel Abalo. "Effects of coffee and its components on the gastrointestinal tract and the brain-gut axis." *Nutrients* 13, no. 1 (December 2020):88. doi:10.3390/nu13010088.

Koochakpoor, Glareh, Asma Salari-Moghaddam, Ammar H. Keshteli, Ahmed Esmaillzadeh, Peyman Adibi. "Association of coffee and caffeine intake with irritable bowel syndrome in adults." *Frontiers in Nutrition* 15, no. 8 (June 2021):632469. doi: 10.3389/fnut.2021.632469.

Mitchell, Diane C., Carol A. Knight, Jon Hockenberry, Robyn Teplansky, Terryl J. Hartman. "Beverage caffeine intakes in the U.S." *Food and Chemical Toxicology* 63 (January 2014):136–142. doi: 10.1016/j.fct.2013.10.042.

National Learning Consortium. "Shared decision making." December 2013. www.healthit.gov/sites/default/files/nlc_shared_decision_making_fact _sheet.pdf.

Reding, Kerryn W., Kevin C. Cain, Monica E. Jarrett, Margaret D. Eugenio, Margaret M. Heitkemper. "Relationship between patterns of alcohol consumption and gastrointestinal symptoms among patients with irritable bowel syndrome." *American Journal of Gastroenterology* 108, no. 2 (February 2013):270–276. doi: 10.1038/ajg.2012.414.

Rej, Anupam, David S. Sanders, Christian C. Shaw, Rachel Buckle, Nick Trott, Anurag Agrawal, Imran Aziz. "Efficacy and acceptability of dietary therapies in non-constipated irritable bowel syndrome: a randomized trial of traditional dietary advice, the low FODMAP diet, and the gluten-free diet." *Clinical Gastroenterology and Hepatology* 20, no. 12 (December 2022):2876–2887.e15. doi: 10.1016/j.cgh.2022.02.045.

Simrén, Magnus, P. Agerforz, E. S. Björnsson, H. Abrahamsson. "Nutrient-dependent enhancement of rectal sensitivity in irritable bowel syndrome (IBS)." *Journal of Neurogastroenterology and Motility* 19, no. 1 (January 2007):20–29. doi: 10.1111/j.1365-2982.2006.00849.x.

Simrén, Magnus, A. Månsson, A. Langkilde, J. Svedlund, H. Abrahamsson, U. Bengtsson, E. Björnsson. "Food-related gastrointestinal symptoms in the irritable bowel syndrome." *Digestion* 63, no. 2 (2001):108–115. doi: 10.1159/000051878.

CHAPTER 6

Biesiekierski, J. R., O. Rosella, R. Rose, K. Liels, J. S. Barrett, S. J. Shepherd, P. R. Gibson, et al. "Quantification of fructans, galacto-oligosaccharides and other short-chain carbohydrates in processed grains and cereals." *Journal of Human Nutrition and Dietetics* 24, no. 2 (April 2011):154–176. doi: 10.1111/j.1365-277X.2010.01139.x.

Diet vs. Disease. "'Eat This, Not That' FODMAPS food list." Last updated September 3, 2023. www.dietvsdisease.org/low-fodmaps-food-list/?gad=1&gclid=CjwKCAjw6eWnBhAKEiwADpnw9vCPGLRIKNRP5HEMi5I29y7HRJ_wBuYKRV3-gUkdwQMfyvD5LFNWhxoCTjsQAvD_BwE.

FODMAP Everyday. "Low FODMAP foods list." Accessed September 10, 2023. www.fodmapeveryday.com/wp-content/uploads/2018/01/FODMAP-Everyday-Low-FODMAP-Foods-List-Full-Color-1.13.18.pdf.

Muir, Jane G., Rosemary Rose, Ourania Rosella, K. Liels, Jacqueline S. Barrett, Susan J. Shepherd, Peter R. Gibson. "Measurement of short-chain carbohydrates in common Australian vegetables and fruits by high-performance liquid chromatography (HPLC)." *Journal of Agricultural and Food Chemistry* 57, no. 2 (January 2009):554–565. doi: 10.1021/jf802700e.

Muir, Jane G., Susan J. Shepherd, Ourania Rosella, Rosemary Rose, Jacqueline S. Barrett, Peter R. Gibson. "Fructan and free fructose content of common Australian vegetables and fruit." *Journal of Agricultural and Food Chemistry* 55, no. 16 (August 2007):6619–6627. doi: 10.1021/jf070623x.

Palmer, Sharon. "How do I get vitamin B12 on a vegan diet?," March 18, 2021. https://sharonpalmer.com/how-to-get-vitamin-b12-on-a-vegan-diet/.

Palmer, Sharon. "How do I get vitamin D on a plant-based diet?," March 26, 2017. https://sharonpalmer.com/ask-sharon-how-do-i-get-vitamin-d-on-a -plant-based-diet/.

Varney, Jane, Jacqueline Barrett, Kate Scarlata, Patsy Catsos, Peter R. Gibson, Jane G. Muir. "FODMAPs: food composition, defining cutoff values and international application." *Journal of Gastroenterology and Hepatology* 32, Suppl. 1 (March 2017):53–61. doi: 10.1111/jgh.13698.

Winther, Gudrun, Betina M. Pyndt Jørgensen, Betina Elfving, Denis S. Nielsen, Pernille Kihl, Sten Lund, Dorte B. Sørensen, et al. "Dietary magnesium deficiency alters gut microbiota and leads to depressive-like behaviour." *Acta Neuropsychiatrica* 27, no. 3 (June 2015):168–176. doi: 10.1017/neu.2015.7.

CHAPTER 7

Bruce, Lauren J., Lina A. Ricciardelli. "A systematic review of the psychosocial correlates of intuitive eating among adult women." *Appetite* 96 (January 2016):454–472. doi: 10.1016/j.appet.2015.10.012.

Burton Murray, Helen, Samantha Calabrese. "Identification and management of eating disorders (including ARFID) in GI patients." *Gastroenterology Clinics of North America* 51, no. 4 (December 2022):765–783. doi:10.1016/j .gtc.2022.07.004.

Cottrell, Damon B., Jeffrey Williams. "Eating disorders in men." *Nurse Practitioner* 41, no. 9 (September 2016):49–55. doi: 10.1097/01 .NPR.0000490392.51227.a2.

Galmiche, Marie, Pierre Déchelotte, Gregory Lambert, Maria P. Tavolacci. "Prevalence of eating disorders over the 2000–2018 period: a systematic literature review." *American Journal of Clinical Nutrition* 109, no. 5 (May 2019):1402–1413. doi: 10.1093/ajcn/nqy342.

Hazzard, Vivienne M., Susan E. Telke, Melissa Simone, Lisa M. Anderson, Nicole I. Larson, Dianne Neumark-Sztainer. "Intuitive eating longitudinally predicts better psychological health and lower use of disordered eating behaviors: findings from EAT 2010–2018." *Eating and Weight Disorders* 26, no. 1 (February 2021):287–294. doi: 10.1007/s40519-020-00852-4.

National Library of Medicine. "Table 22: DSM-IV to DSM-5 avoidant/ restrictive food intake disorder comparison." June 2016. www.ncbi.nlm .nih.gov/books/NBK519712/table/ch3.t18/.

Nicholas, Julia K., Miranda A. L. van Tilburg, Ilana Pilato, Savanna Erwin, Alannah Rivera-Cancel, Lindsay Ives, Marsha D. Marcus, et al. "The diagnosis of avoidant restrictive food intake disorder in the presence of gastrointestinal disorders: opportunities to define shared mechanisms of symptom expression." *International Journal of Eating Disorders* 54, no. 6 (June 2021):995–1008. doi: 10.1002/eat.23536.

Riehl, Megan E., Kate Scarlata. "Understanding disordered eating risks in patients with gastrointestinal conditions." *Journal of the Academy of Nutrition and Dietetics* 122, no. 3 (2022):491–499. doi: 10.1016/j.jand.2021.03.001.

Sidani, Jaine E., Ariel Shensa, Beth Hoffman, Janel Hanmer, Brian A. Primack. "The association between social media use and eating concerns among US young adults." *Journal of the Academy of Nutrition and Dietetics* 116, no. 9 (September 2016):1465–1472. doi: 10.1016/j.jand.2016.03.021.

Tribole, Evelyn, Elyse Resch. *Intuitive Eating*, 4th ed. (New York: St. Martin's, 2020).

Tuck, Caroline J., Nessmah Sultan, Matilda Tonkovic, Jessica R. Biesiekierski. "Orthorexia nervosa is a concern in gastroenterology: a scoping review." *Journal of Neurogastroenterology and Motility* 34, no. 8 (August 2022):e14427. doi: 10.1111/nmo.14427.

van Hoeken, Daphne, Hans W. Hoek. "Review of the burden of eating disorders: mortality, disability, costs, quality of life, and family burden." *Current Opinion in Psychiatry* 33, no. 6 (November 2020):521–527. doi: 10.1097/YCO.0000000000000641.

CHAPTER 8

Anderson, Jason R., Ian Carroll, M. Andrea Azcarate-Peril, Amber D. Rochette, Leslie J. Heinberg, Christine Peat, Kristine Steffen, et al. "A preliminary examination of gut microbiota, sleep, and cognitive flexibility in healthy older adults." *Sleep Medicine* 38 (October 2017):104–107. doi: 10.1016/j.sleep.2017.07.018.

Bäckhed, Fredrik, Claire M. Fraser, Yehuda Ringel, Mary E. Sanders, R. Balfour Sartor, Philip M. Sherman, James Versalovic, et al. "Defining a healthy human gut microbiome: current concepts, future directions, and clinical applications." *Cell Host and Microbe* 12, no. 5 (November 2012):611–622. doi: 10.1016/j.chom.2012.10.012.

Centers for Disease Control and Prevention. "Tips for better sleep." September 13, 2022. www.cdc.gov/sleep/about_sleep/sleep_hygiene.html.

Chedid, Victor, Sameer Dhalla, John O. Clarke, Bani C. Roland, Kerry B. Dunbar, Joyce Koh, Edmundo Justino, et al. "Herbal therapy is equivalent to rifaximin for the treatment of small intestinal bacterial overgrowth." *Global Advances in Health and Medicine* 3, no. 3 (May 2014):16–24. doi: 10.7453/gahmj.2014.019.

Dimidi, Eirini, Selina R. Cox, Megan Rossi, Kevin Whelan. "Fermented foods: definitions and characteristics, impact on the gut microbiota and effects on gastrointestinal health and disease." *Nutrients* 11, no. 8 (August 2019):1806. doi: 10.3390/nu11081806.

Ducrotté, Philippe, Prabha Sawant, Venkataraman Jayanthi. "Clinical trial: *Lactobacillus plantarum* 299v (DSM 9843) improves symptoms of irritable bowel syndrome." *World Journal of Gastroenterology* 18, no. 30 (August 2012):4012–4018. doi: 10.3748/wjg.v18.i30.4012.

Ghoshal, Uday C., Ujjala Ghoshal. "Small intestinal bacterial overgrowth and other intestinal disorders." *Gastroenterology Clinics of North America* 46, no. 1 (March 2017):103–120. doi: 10.1016/j.gtc.2016.09.008.

Ghoshal, Uday C., Abhimanyu Nehra, Akash Mathur, Sushmita Rai. "A meta-analysis on small intestinal bacterial overgrowth in patients with different subtypes of irritable bowel syndrome." *Journal of Gastroenterology and Hepatology* 35, no. 6 (June 2020):922–931. doi: 10.1111/jgh.14938.

Ghoshal, Uday C., Deepakshi Srivastava. "Irritable bowel syndrome and small intestinal bacterial overgrowth: meaningful association or unnecessary hype?," *World Journal of Gastroenterology* 20, no. 10 (March 2014):2482–2491. doi: 10.3748/wjg.v20.i10.2482.

Ishaque, Shamsuddin, S. M. Khosruzzaman, Dewan S. Ahmed, Mukesh P. Sah. "A randomized placebo-controlled clinical trial of a multi-strain probiotic formulation (Bio-Kult®) in the management of diarrhea-predominant irritable bowel syndrome." *BMC Gastroenterology* 18, no. 1 (May 2018):71. doi: 10.1186/s12876-018-0788-9.

Lacy, Brian E., Mark Pimentel, Darren M. Brenner, William D. Chey, Laurie A. Keefer, Millie D. Long, Baha Moshiree. "ACG clinical guideline: management of irritable bowel syndrome." *American Journal of Gastroenterology* 116, no. 1 (January 2021):17–44. doi.10.14309/ajg.0000000000001036.

Leite, Gabriela, Walter Morales, Stacy Weitsman, Shreya Celly, Gonzalo Parodi, Ruchi Mathur, Gillian M. Barlow, et al. "The duodenal microbiome is altered in small intestinal bacterial overgrowth." *PLoS One* 15, no. 7 (July 2020):e0234906. doi: 10.1371/journal.pone.0234906.

Phan, Joann, Divya Nair, Suneer Jain, Thibaut Montagne, Demi V. Flores, Andre Nguyen, Summer Dietsche, et al. "Alterations in gut microbiome composition and function in irritable bowel syndrome and increased probiotic abundance with daily supplementation." *mSystems* 6, no. 6 (December 2021):e0121521. doi: 10.1128/mSystems.01215-21.

Pimentel, Mark, Ava Hosseini, Christine Chang, Ruchi Mathur, Mohammed Rashid, Rashin Sedighi, Halley Fowler, et al. "Fr248 exhaled hydrogen sulfide is increased in patients with diarrhea: results of a novel collection and breath testing device." *Gastroenterology* 160 (2021):S-278. doi: 10.1016/S0016- 5085(21)01391-3.

Pimentel, Mark, Richard J. Saad, Millie D. Long, Satish S. C. Rao. "ACG clinical guideline: small intestinal bacterial overgrowth." *American Journal of Gastroenterology* 115, no. 2 (February 2020):165–178. doi: 10.14309/ajg.0000000000000501.

Rao, Satish S. C., Jigar Bhagatwala. "Small intestinal bacterial overgrowth: clinical features and therapeutic management." *Clinical and*

Translational Gastroenterology 10, no. 10 (October 2019):e00078. doi: 10.14309/ctg.0000000000000078.

Rezaie, Ali, Michelle Buresi, Anthony Lembo, Henry Lin, Richard McCallum, Satish Rao, Max Schmulson, et al. "Hydrogen- and methane-based breath testing in gastrointestinal disorders: the North American consensus." *American Journal of Gastroenterology* 112, no. 5 (May 2017):775–784. doi: 10.1038/ajg.2017.46.

Riccio, Paola, and Rocco Rossano. "The human gut microbiota is neither an organ nor a commensal." *FEBS Letters* 594, no. 20 (2020):3262–3271. doi: 10.1002/1873-3468.13946.

Rinninella, Emanuele, Pauline Raoul, Marco Cintoni, Francesco Franceschi, Giacinto Abele, Donato Miggiano, Antonio Gasbarrini, Marina C. Mele. "What is the healthy gut microbiota composition? A changing ecosystem across age, environment, diet, and diseases." *Microorganisms* 7, no. 1 (January 2019):14. doi: 10.3390/microorganisms7010014.

Scarlata, Kate. "Small intestinal bacterial overgrowth: what to do when unwelcome microbes invade." *Today's Dietitian* 13, no. 4 (2011):46.

Shah, Ayesha, Nicholas J. Talley, Mike Jones, Bradley J. Kendall, Natasha Koloski, Marjorie M. Walker, Mark Morrison, et al. "Small intestinal bacterial overgrowth in irritable bowel syndrome: a systematic review and meta-analysis of case-control studies." *American Journal of Gastroenterology* 115, no. 2 (February 2020):190–201. doi: 10.14309/ajg.0000000000000504.

Skokovic-Sunjic, Dragana. "Clinical guide to probiotic products available in the USA." AEProbio, last modified January 2023. https://usprobiotic guide.com.

Skrzydło-Radomańska, Barbara, Beata Prozorow-Król, Halina Cichoż-Lach, Emilia Majsiak, Joanna B. Bierła, Ewelina Kanarek, Agnieszka Sowińska, et al. "The effectiveness and safety of multi-strain probiotic preparation in patients with diarrhea-predominant irritable bowel syndrome: a randomized controlled study." *Nutrients* 13, no. 3 (February 2021):756. doi: 10.3390/nu13030756.

Smith, Robert P., Cole Easson, Sarah M. Lyle, Ritishka Kapoor, Chase P. Donnelly, Eileen J. Davidson, Esha Parikh, et al. "Gut microbiome diversity is associated with sleep physiology in humans." *PLoS One* 14, no. 10 (October 2019):e0222394. doi: 10.1371/journal.pone.0222394.

Takahashi, Toku. "Mechanism of interdigestive migrating motor complex." *Journal of Neurogastroenterology and Motility* 18, no. 3 (July 2012):246–257. doi: 10.5056/jnm.2012.18.3.246.

Takakura, Will, and Mark Pimentel. "Small intestinal bacterial overgrowth and irritable bowel syndrome: an update." *Frontiers in Psychiatry* 11 (July 2020):664. doi: 10.3389/fpsyt.2020.00664.

Trio-Smart. "Is Trio-Smart right for you?," Accessed August 21, 2023. www.triosmartbreath.com/.

Wastyk, Hannah C., Gabriela K. Fragiadakis, Dalia Perelman, Dylan Dahan, Bryan D. Merrill, Feiqiao B. Yu, Madeline Topf, et al. "Gut-microbiota-targeted diets modulate human immune status." *Cell* 184, no. 16 (August 2021):4137–4153.e14. doi: 10.1016/j.cell.2021.06.019.

Whole Body Health Physical Therapy. "Massage for your gut!," November 3, 2014. www.wholebodyhealth-pt.com/wbhptblog/massage-for-your-gut.

CHAPTER 9

Aucoin, Monique, Laura LaChance, Umadevi Naidoo, Daniella Remy, Tanisha Shekdar, Negin Sayar, Valentina Cardozo, et al. "Diet and anxiety: a scoping review." *Nutrients* 13, no. 12 (December 2021):4418. doi: 10.3390/nu13124418.

Barba, Elizabeth, Emanuel Burri, Anna Accarino, Daniel Cisternas, Sergi Quiroga, Eva Monclus, Isabel Navazo, et al. "Abdominothoracic mechanisms of functional abdominal distension and correction by biofeedback." *Gastroenterology* 148, no. 4 (2015):732–739. doi: 10.1053/j.gastro.2014.12.006.

Bellini, Massimo, Sara Tonarelli, Federico Barracca, Francesco Rettura, Andrea Pancetti, Linda Ceccarelli, Angelo Ricchiuti, et al. "Chronic constipation: is a nutritional approach reasonable?," *Nutrients* 13, no. 10 (September 2021):3386. doi: 10.3390/nu13103386.

Bharucha, Adil E., Subhankar Chakraborty, Christopher D. Sletten. "Common functional gastroenterological disorders associated with abdominal pain." *Mayo Clinical Proceedings* 91, no. 8 (August 2016):1118–1132. doi: 10.1016/j.mayocp.2016.06.003.

Bharucha, Adil E., and Brian E. Lacy. "Mechanisms, evaluation, and management of chronic constipation." *Gastroenterology* 158, no. 5 (April 2020):1232–1249.e3. doi: 10.1053/j.gastro.2019.12.034.

Brenner, Darren M., and Brian E. Lacy. "Antispasmodics for chronic abdominal pain: analysis of North American treatment options." *American Journal of Gastroenterology* 116, no. 8 (August 2021):1587–1600. doi: 10.14309/ajg.0000000000001266.

Cappello, G., M. Spezzaferro, L. Grossi, L. Manzoli, L. Marzio. "Peppermint oil (Mintoil®) in the treatment of irritable bowel syndrome: a prospective double blind placebo-controlled randomized trial." *Digestive and Liver Disease* 39, no. 6 (2007):530–536. doi: 10.1016/j.dld.2007.02.006.

Carrasco-Labra, Alonso, Lyubov Lytvyn, Yngve Falck-Ytter, Christina M. Surawicz, William D. Chey. "AGA technical review on the evaluation of functional diarrhea and diarrhea-predominant irritable bowel syndrome in adults (IBS-D)." *Gastroenterology* 157, no. 3 (September 2019):859–880. doi: 10.1053/j.gastro.2019.06.014.

Chang, Lin, Shahnaz Sultan, Anthony Lembo, G. Nicholas Verne, Walter Smalley, Joel J. Heidelbaugh. "AGA clinical practice guideline on the pharmacological management of irritable bowel syndrome with constipation." *Gastroenterology* 163, no. 1 (July 2022):118–136. doi: 10.1053/j.gastro.2022.04.016.

Chey, William D., Jana G. Hashash, Laura Manning, Lin Chang. "AGA clinical practice update on the role of diet in irritable bowel syndrome: expert review." *Gastroenterology* 162, no. 6 (May 2022):1737–1745.e5. doi: 10.1053/j.gastro.2021.12.248.

Del Toro-Barbosa, Mariano, Alejandra Hurtado-Romero, Luis Eduardo Garcia-Amezquita, Tomas García-Cayuela. "Psychobiotics: mechanisms of action, evaluation methods and effectiveness in applications with food products." *Nutrients* 12, no. 12 (December 2020):3896. doi: 10.3390/nu12123896.

Dimidi, Eirini, S. Mark Scott, Kevin Whelan. "Probiotics and constipation: mechanisms of action, evidence for effectiveness and utilisation by patients and healthcare professionals." *Proceedings of the Nutrition Society* 78, no. 1 (February 2020):147–157. doi: 10.1017/S0029665119000934. Erratum in: *Proceedings of the Nutrition Society* 78, no. 1 (February 2020):170.

Drossman, Douglas A., Brenda B. Toner, William E. Whitehead, Nicholas E. Diamant, Chris B. Dalton, Susan Duncun, Shelagh Emmott, et al. "Cognitive-behavioral therapy versus education and desipramine versus placebo for moderate to severe functional bowel disorders." *Gastroenterology* 125, no. 1 (2003):19–31. doi:10.1016/s0016-5085(03)00669-3.

Fragkos, Konstantinos C., Natalia Zárate-Lopez, Christos C. Frangos. "What about clonidine for diarrhoea? A systematic review and meta-analysis of its effect in humans." *Therapeutic Advances in Gastroenterology* 9, no. 3 (May 2016):282–301. doi: 10.1177/1756283X15625586.

Greenberg, Jeffrey, Anderson A. Tesfazion, Christopher S. Robinson. "Screening, diagnosis, and treatment of depression." *Military Medicine* 177, no. 8 (August 2012):60–66. doi: 10.7205/milmed-d-12-00102.

Iovino, Paola, Maria C. Neri, Lucia D'Alba, Antonella Santonicola, Giuseppe Chiarioni. "Pelvic floor biofeedback is an effective treatment for severe bloating in disorders of gut-brain interaction with outlet dysfunction." *Journal of Neurogastroenterology and Motility* 34, no. 5 (May 2022):e14264. doi: 10.1111/nmo.14264.

Jagielski, Christina, Jessica Naftaly, Megan Riehl. "Providing trauma-informed care during anorectal evaluation." *Current Gastroenterology Reports* 25, no. 9 (August 2023): 204–211. doi: 10.1007/s11894-023-00879-4.

Jiang, X., G. Locke, R. Choung, A. Zinsmeister, C. Schleck, N. Talley. "Prevalence and risk factors for abdominal bloating and visible distention: a population-based study." *Gut* 57, no. 6 (2008):756–763. doi: 10.1136/gut.2007.142810.

Komericki, P., M. Akkilic-Materna, T. Strimitzer, K. Weyermair, H. F. Hammer, W. Aberer. "Oral xylose isomerase decreases breath hydrogen excretion and improves gastrointestinal symptoms in fructose malabsorption:

a double-blind, placebo-controlled study." *Alimentary Pharmacology and Therapeutics* 36, no. 10 (November 2012):980–987. doi: 10.1111/apt.12057.

Lacy, Brian E., Mark Pimentel, Darren M. Brenner, William D. Chey, Laurie A. Keefer, Millie D. Long, Baharak Moshiree. "ACG clinical guideline: management of irritable bowel syndrome." *American Journal of Gastroenterology* 116, no. 1 (January 2021):17–44. doi: 10.14309 /ajg.0000000000001036.

Lakhoo, Krutika, Christopher V. Almario, Carine Khalil, Brennan M. R. Spiegel. "Prevalence and characteristics of abdominal pain in the United States." *Clinical Gastroenterology and Hepatology* 19, no. 9 (September 2021):1864–1872.e5. doi: 10.1016/j.cgh.2020.06.065.

Lembo, Anthony, Shahnaz Sultan, Lin Chang, Joel J. Heidelbaugh, Walter Smalley, G. Nicholas Verne. "AGA clinical practice guideline on the pharmacological management of irritable bowel syndrome with diarrhea." *Gastroenterology* 163, no. 1 (July 2022):137–151. doi: 10.1053/j .gastro.2022.04.017.

Lin, Hao, Gingqing Guo, Zhiyong Wen, Songlin Tan, Jie Chen, Lijian Lin, Pengcheng Chen, et al. "The multiple effects of fecal microbiota transplantation on diarrhea-predominant irritable bowel syndrome (IBS-D) patients with anxiety and depression behaviors." *Microbial Cell Factories* 20, no. 1 (December 2021):233. doi: 10.1186/s12934-021-01720-1.

Liu, Baoyan, Jiani Wu, Shiyan Yan, Kehua Zhou, Liyun He, Jianqiao Fang, Wenbin Fu, et al. "Electroacupuncture vs. prucalopride for severe chronic constipation: a multicenter, randomized, controlled, noninferiority trial." *American Journal of Gastroenterology* 116, no. 5 (May 2021):1024–1035. doi: 10.14309/ajg.0000000000001050.

Liu, Jenn-Hua, Gran-Hum Chen, Hong-Zen Yeh, Chin-Kuen Huang, Sek-Kwong Poon. "Enteric-coated peppermint-oil capsules in the treatment of irritable bowel syndrome: a prospective, randomized trial." *Journal of Gastroenterology* 32, no. 6 (1997):765–768. doi: 10.1007/BF02936952.

Malagelada, Juan, Anna Accarino, Fernando Azpiroz. "Bloating and abdominal distension: old misconceptions and current knowledge." *American Journal of Gastroenterology* 112, no. 8 (2017):1221–1231. doi: 10.1038 /ajg.2017.129.

Mari, Amir, Fadi Abu Backer, Mahmud Mahamid, Hana Amara, Dan Carter, Doron Boltin, Ram Dickman. "Bloating and abdominal distension: clinical approach and management." *Advances in Therapy* 36, no. 5 (May 2019):1075–1084. doi: 10.1007/s12325-019-00924-7.

Martoni, Christopher J., Shalini Srivastava, Gregory J. Leyer. "Lactobacillus acidophilus DDS-1 and Bifidobacterium lactis UABla-12 improve abdominal pain severity and symptomology in irritable bowel syndrome: randomized controlled trial." *Nutrients* 12, no. 2 (January 2020):363. doi: 10.3390/nu12020363.

Qi, Ling-Yu, Jing-Wen Yang, Shi-Yan Yan, Jian-Feng Tu, Yan-Fen She, Ying Li, Li-Li Chi, et al. "Acupuncture for the treatment of diarrhea-predominant irritable bowel syndrome: a pilot randomized clinical trial." *JAMA Network Open* 5, no. 12 (December 2022):e2248817. doi: 10.1001/jamanetworkopen.2022.48817.

Quigley, Eamonn M. M., Josepha A. Murray, Mark Pimentel. "AGA clinical practice update on small intestinal bacterial overgrowth: expert review." *Gastroenterology* 159, no. 4 (October 2020):1526–1532. doi: 10.1053/j.gastro.2020.06.090.

Rao, Satish S. C., Eamonn M. M. Quigley, William D. Chey, Amol Sharma, Anthony J. Lembo. "Randomized placebo-controlled phase 3 trial of vibrating capsule for chronic constipation." *Gastroenterology* 164, no. 7 (June 2023):1202–1210.e6. doi: 10.1053/j.gastro.2023.02.013.

Rose, Matthias, and Janine Devine. "Assessment of patient-reported symptoms of anxiety." *Dialogues in Clinical Neuroscience* 16, no. 2 (June 2014):197–211. doi: 10.31887/DCNS.2014.16.2/mrose.

Schiller, Lawrence R., Darrell S. Pardi, Joseph H. Sellin. "Chronic diarrhea: diagnosis and management." *Clinical Gastroenterology and Hepatology* 15, no. 2 (February 2017):182–193.e3. doi: 10.1016/j.cgh.2016.07.028.

Schmulson, Max, and Lin Chang. "Review article: the treatment of functional abdominal bloating and distension." *Alimentary Pharmacology and Therapeutics* 33, no. 10 (2011):1071–1086. doi: 10.1111/j.1365-2036.2011.04637.x.

Serra, Jordi. "Management of bloating." *Journal of Neurogastroenterology and Motility* 34, no. 3 (March 2022):e14333. doi: 10.1111/nmo.14333.

Spiegel, Brennan M. R., Omer Liran, Rebecca Gale, Carine Khalil, Katherine Makaroff, Robert Chernoff, Tiffany Raber, et al. "Qualitative validation of a novel VR program for irritable bowel syndrome: a VR1 study." *American Journal of Gastroenterology* 117, no. 3 (March 2022):495–500. doi: 10.14309/ajg.0000000000001641.

Tack, J., D. Broekaert, B. Fischler, L. Van Oudenhove, A. M. Gevers, J. Janssens. "A controlled crossover study of the selective serotonin reuptake inhibitor citalopram in irritable bowel syndrome." *Gut* 55, no. 8 (August 2006):1095–1103. doi: 10.1136/gut.2005.077503.

Zhou, Jing, Yan Liu, Kehua Zhou, Baoyan Liu, Tongsheng Su, Weiming Wang, Zhishun Liu. "Electroacupuncture for women with chronic severe functional constipation: subgroup analysis of a randomized controlled trial." *Biomed Research International* 2019 (January 2019):7491281. doi: 10.1155/2019/7491281.

CHAPTER 10

Ashtari, Sara, Hadis Najafimehr, Mohamad A. Pourhoseingholi, Kamran Rostami, Hamid Asadzadeh-Aghdaei, Mohammad Rostami-Nejad, Mostafa R. Tavirani, et al. "Prevalence of celiac disease in low and high risk population in Asia–Pacific region: a systematic review and meta-analysis." *Scientific Reports* 11, no. 1 (December 2021):2383. doi: 10.1038/s41598-021-82023-8.

Brown, Benjamin I. "Does irritable bowel syndrome exist? Identifiable and treatable causes of associated symptoms suggest it may not." *Gastrointestinal Disorders* 1, no. 3 (2019):314–340. doi: 10.3390/gidisord1030027.

Caio, Giacomo, Umberto Volta, Anna Sapone, Daniel A. Leffler, Roberto De Giorgio, Carlo Catassi, Alessio Fasano. "Celiac disease: a comprehensive current review." *BMC Medicine* 12, no. 1 (December 2019):142. doi: 10.1186/s12916-019-1380-z.

Camilleri, Michael. "Bile acid diarrhea: prevalence, pathogenesis, and therapy." *Gut and Liver* 9, no. 3 (May 2015):332–339. doi: 10.5009/gnl14397.

Catassi, Carlo, Debby Kryszak, Bushra Bhatti, Craig Sturgeon, Kathy Helzlsouer, Sandra L. Clipp, Daniel Gelfond, et al. "Natural history of celiac disease autoimmunity in a USA cohort followed since 1974." *Annals of Medicine* 42, no. 7 (October 2010):530–538. doi: 10.3109/07853890.2010.514285.

Centers for Disease Control and Prevention. "Parasites: giardia." Last reviewed February 26, 2021. www.cdc.gov/parasites/giardia/general-info .html.

Centers for Disease Control and Prevention. "People with IBD have more chronic diseases." April 15, 2022. www.cdc.gov/ibd/features/IBD-more -chronic-diseases.html.

Centers for Disease Control and Prevention. "Waterborne disease and outbreak surveillance reporting." December 12, 2022. www.cdc.gov /healthywater/surveillance/giardiasis/giardiasis-2019.html.

Chin, Russell L., Norman Latov, Peter H. R. Green, Thomas H. Brannagan, Armin Alaedini, Howard Sander. "Neurologic complications of celiac disease." *Journal of Clinical Neuromuscular Disease* 5, no. 3 (March 2004):129–137. doi: 10.1097/00131402-200403000-00004.

Crohn's and Colitis Foundation. "How is IBD diagnosed?," Accessed September 8, 2023. www.crohnscolitisfoundation.org/what-is-ibd/diagnosing -ibd.

Fasano, Alessio, and Carlo Catassi. "Clinical practice: celiac disease." *New England Journal of Medicine* 367, no. 25 (December 2012):2419–2426. doi: 10.1056/NEJMcp1113994.

GBD 2017 Inflammatory Bowel Disease Collaborators. "The global, regional, and national burden of inflammatory bowel disease in 195 countries and territories, 1990–2017: a systematic analysis for the Global Burden of Disease Study 2017." *Lancet Gastroenterology and Hepatology* 5, no. 1 (January 2020):17–30. doi: 10.1016/S2468-1253(19)30333-4.

Hadjivassiliou, Marios, Iain D. Croall, Panagiotis Zis, Ptolemaios G. Sarrigiannis, David S. Sanders, Pascale Aeschlimann, Richard A. Grunewald, et al. "Neurologic deficits in patients with newly diagnosed celiac disease are frequent and linked with autoimmunity to transglutaminase 6." *Clinical*

Gastroenterology and Hepatology 17, no. 13 (December 2019):2678–2686.e2. doi:10.1016/j.cgh.2019.03.014.

Halpin, Stephen J., and Alexander C. Ford. "Prevalence of symptoms meeting criteria for irritable bowel syndrome in inflammatory bowel disease: systematic review and meta-analysis." *American Journal of Gastroenterology* 107, no. 10 (2012):1474–1482. doi: 10.1038/ajg.2012.260.

Hanevik, Kurt, Vernesa Dizdar, Nina Langeland, Trygve Hausken. "Development of functional gastrointestinal disorders after *Giardia lamblia* infection." *BMC Gastroenterology* 9 (2007):27. doi: 10.1186/1471-230X-9-27.

Jacob, Ralf, Klaus-Peter Zimmer, Jacques Schmitz, Hassan Y. Naim. "Congenital sucrase-isomaltase deficiency arising from cleavage and secretion of a mutant form of the enzyme." *Journal of Clinical Investigation* 106, no. 2 (July 2000):281–287. doi: 10.1172/JCI9677.

Jericho, Hilary, Naire Sansotta, Stefano Guandalini. "Extraintestinal manifestations of celiac disease: effectiveness of the gluten-free diet." *Journal of Pediatric Gastroenterology and Nutrition* 65, no. 1 (2017):75–79. doi: 10.1097/MPG.0000000000001420.

Kalra, Neetu, Anuska Mukerjee, Shreya Sinha, Vaishnavi Muralidhar, Yeliz Serin, Aadhya Tiwari, Anil K. Verma. "Current updates on the association between celiac disease and cancer, and the effects of the gluten-free diet for modifying the risk (review)." *International Journal of Functional Nutrition* 3, no. 1 (January 2022). doi: 10.3892/ijfn.2022.25.

Kårhus, Line L., Tea Skaaby, Janne Petersen, Anja L. Madsen, Betina H. Thuesen, Peter Schwarz, Juri J. Rumessen, et al. "Long-term consequences of undiagnosed celiac seropositivity." *American Journal of Gastroenterology* 115, no. 10 (October 2020):1681–1688. doi: 10.14309/ajg.0000000000000737.

Moshiree, Baha, Joel J. Heidelbaugh, Gregory S. Sayuk. "A narrative review of irritable bowel syndrome with diarrhea: a primer for primary care providers." *Advances in Therapy* 39, no. 9 (September 2022):4003–4020. doi: 10.1007/s12325-022-02224-z.

Olmos, Juan I., Maria M. Piskorz, Nestor Litwin, Sara Schaab, Adriana Tevez, Gladys Bravo-Velez, Tatiana Uehara, et al. "Exocrine pancreatic insufficiency is undiagnosed in some patients with diarrhea-predominant irritable bowel syndrome using the Rome IV criteria." *Digestive Diseases and Sciences* 67, no. 12 (December 2022):5666–5675. doi: 10.1007/s10620-022-07568-8.

Paez, Marco A., Anna Maria Gramelspacher, James Sinacore, Laura Winterfield, Mukund Venu. "Delay in diagnosis of celiac disease in patients without gastrointestinal complaints." *American Journal of Medicine* 130, no. 11 (November 2017):1318–1323. doi: 10.1016/j.amjmed.2017.05.027

Pimentel, Mark, Richard J. Saad, Millie D. Long, Satish S. C. Rao. "ACG clinical guideline: small intestinal bacterial overgrowth." *American*

Journal of Gastroenterology 115, no. 2 (February 2020):165–178. doi: 10.14309 /ajg.0000000000000501.

Rao, Satish S. C., and Tanisa Patcharatrakul. "Diagnosis and treatment of dyssynergic defecation." *Journal of Neurogastroenterology and Motility* 22, no. 3 (July 2016):423–435. doi: 10.5056/jnm16060.

Rome Foundation. "Appendix A: Rome IV diagnostic criteria for FGIDs." January 16, 2016. https://theromefoundation.org/rome-iv/rome-iv-criteria/.

Sainsbury, Anita, David S. Sanders, Alexander C. Ford. "Prevalence of irritable bowel syndrome–type symptoms in patients with celiac disease: a meta-analysis." *Clinical Gastroenterology and Hepatology* 11, no. 4 (April 2013):359–365.e1. doi: 10.1016/j.cgh.2012.11.033.

Suares, Nicole C., Alexander C. Ford. "Prevalence of, and risk factors for, chronic idiopathic constipation in the community: systematic review and meta-analysis." *American Journal of Gastroenterology* 106, no. 9 (2011):1582–1591. doi: 10.1038/ajg.2011.164.

Walters, Julian R. F. "Bile acid diarrhoea and FGF19: new views on diagnosis, pathogenesis and therapy." *Nature Reviews Gastroenterology and Hepatology* 11, no. 7 (July 2014):426–434. doi: 10.1038/nrgastro.2014.32.

Wierdsma, Nicolette J., Marian Van Bokhorst-De Van Der Schueren, Marijke Berkenpas, Chris J. J. Mulder, Ad A. Van Bodegraven. "Vitamin and mineral deficiencies are highly prevalent in newly diagnosed celiac disease patients." *Nutrients* 5, no. 10 (September 2013):3975–3992. doi: 10.3390 /nu5103975.

ACKNOWLEDGMENTS

From Kate: To my wonderful husband, Russ, who has been my motivational coach and editorial assistant in writing this book. I am truly grateful for you and for the life we have carved out together. A big thanks to my kids, Chelsea, Kevin, and Brennan, for their amazing support as I have navigated my writing and my incredibly rewarding career. I am most proud and grateful for the unconditional love and care we share in our family of five, which we warmly refer to as "the Scarlata 5." Thank you, Dr. Megan Riehl, for joining forces with me to write this very important book that comprehensively addresses IBS management. I am proud of our work together! And last but never least, thank you to the many people living with IBS, true warriors in my eyes, who have trusted in my care and helped make me a better person and clinician.

From Megan: I am beyond blessed with individuals who touch my life and lift me up. This book is dedicated to you. For my beautiful children, Lucas, Liam, and Olivia, you are my sources of pure joy and love. For my husband, Bobby, your encouragement and support mean everything; without you none of this works! For my parents, you are my steadfast sources of faith and unconditional love. For my Women in GI (WIG) sisters, you are my sources of laughter and brilliance. And for my dear friend Kate, you are the perfect partner on this incredible journey to empower all who read and have inspired this book! I am humbled by the opportunity to be a working mom in a helping profession within a field that positively affects lives every day.

From Kate and Megan, the Mind Your Gut Team: A big thank-you to our talented editor, Renée Sedliar, editorial director at Hachette Go, for believing in us! Thank you to Katie Malm and Kelley Blewster for their talented editing and their attention to detail in making our work shine and for truly understanding the needs of those living with IBS. We would not have had this opportunity without our fabulous literary agent, Marilyn Allen at Allen Literary Agency. Thanks, Marilyn!

We are so grateful for the beautiful Foreword written by our esteemed colleague and friend Dr. William D. Chey, chief of gastroenterology at Michigan Medicine. Dr. Chey is a true physician champion who has amplified the importance of integrative care that includes nutrition and psychological interventions for the management of IBS. He has been an incredible advocate for IBS patients as well as for dietitians and psychologists working in the GI space.

INDEX